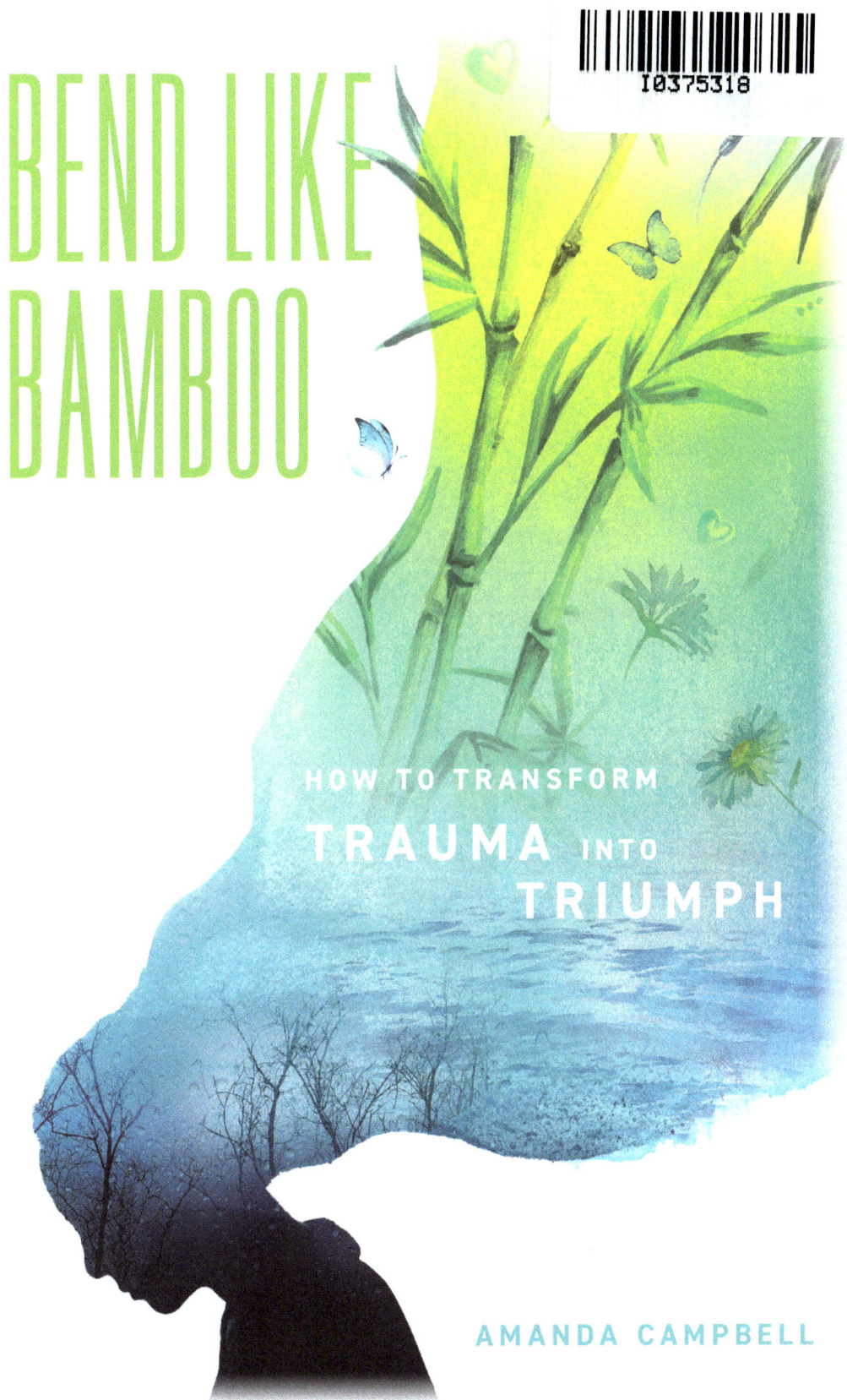

BEND LIKE BAMBOO

HOW TO TRANSFORM TRAUMA INTO TRIUMPH

AMANDA CAMPBELL

First published by Busybird Publishing 2024

Copyright © 2024 Bend Like Bamboo

ISBN:
Paperback: 978-1-922954-85-5
Ebook: 978-1-922954-86-2

This work is copyright. Apart from any use permitted under the *Copyright Act 1968*, no part of this publication may be reproduced, stored in a retrieval system or transmitted in any form or by any means, electronic, mechanical, photocopying, recording or otherwise, without the prior written permission of Amanda Campbell.

The information in this book is based on the author's experiences and opinions. The author and publisher disclaim responsibility for any adverse consequences, which may result from use of the information contained herein. Permission to use any external content has been sought by the author. Any breaches will be rectified in further editions of the book.

Layout and typesetting: Busybird Publishing

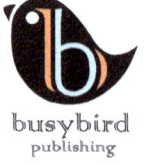

Busybird Publishing
2/118 Para Road
Montmorency, Victoria
Australia 3094
www.busybird.com.au

To Mum, my angel, my guide.

Because you loved me, I know and have experienced the meaning of true unconditional love.

This was the greatest gift. Thank you for your beautiful energy, for showing me the presence and power of spirit and how to access my intuition. Thank you for never judging me, for allowing me to be who I am on my journey, and for your consistent fountain of love that touched me at the deepest level of my soul.

You left this planet on Mother's Day, 9th May 2021, just after midnight, which broke my heart.
Your love was pure, like sunshine and you will forever remain in my heart.

Until we meet again when I cross the other side.
I can't wait to see you, Muma, Billy and Henry again x

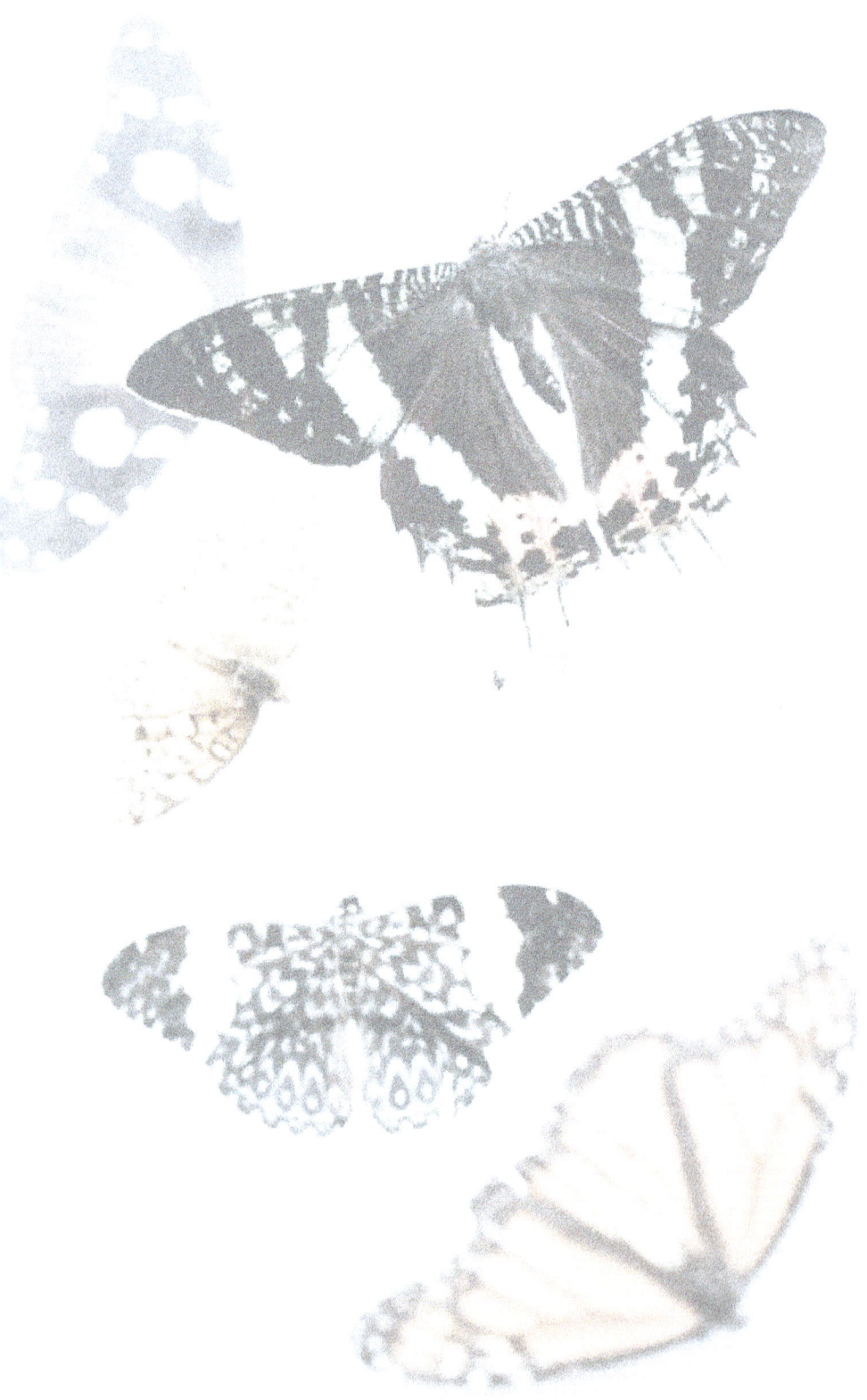

Testimonials

"An inspiring story that shows the power of flexibility and perseverance. Better flexibility, balance and self-care are keys to restoring your vitality. A must read for everyone with a multiple sclerosis diagnosis."

Terry Wahls, MD, IFMCP, Author *The Wahls Protocol A Radical New Way to Treat All Chronic Autoimmune Conditions*

"An inspiring story that shows the power of mindset and self-belief, an excellent guide for those diagnosed with Multiple Sclerosis and Autoimmune Disease."

Damian Brown – Naturopath & Nutritionist

"Learn how to develop a flexible mindset for a better life. This book shares insights from overcoming challenges, gives advice on reducing stress and reaching personal goals. If you want a happier, more resilient life, this book is a valuable guide."

Colleen Callander
Former Sportsgirl CEO & Co Founder of Human Elevation

"Amanda shares her journey living with Multiple Sclerosis and walking again after a left side body paralysis. Her methodological and multi layered approach to her own healing has inspired a book from the heart combining scientific research and practicality. This is a must read for people living with autoimmune disease and anyone going through change, grief or stress in their lives."

Dr Mike Rowan - Osteopath, naturopath, traditional Chinese Acupuncture.

"Amanda shares her story of resilience and possibility, inspiring those diagnosed with MS to rise using their own power of mindset and belief to be the person they have always desired. If you are wanting something more in your life, this book is a must read giving you the power and tools to remain flexible on your journey of recovery!"

Matt Rowe - Author, MS Coach, Symptom Free MS Summit Founder and Host, Reiki and Meditation practitioner and Ironman

Disclaimer

If any information that you read triggers uncomfortable feelings for you, I highly recommend you explore them further for yourself. Sit with them with a flexible mindset, and consider reaching out for support alongside a therapist or practitioner that resonates with you.

The advice in this book is not intended to replace medical care. It is to empower you to believe in yourself on your journey and to investigate what may be causing you stress in areas you may not have considered before. I suggest that you empower yourself to do your own research on how to maximise your own recovery, accompanied by medical advice.

The information in this book is general information and should not be used to diagnose or treat a health problem or disease. Do not use the information found in this book as a substitute for professional healthcare advice. Any information you find in this book, or on external sites which are linked to this book, should be verified with your professional healthcare provider. Amanda Campbell does not make any representation or warranty (express or implied) as to the accuracy or completeness of the information set out in this book and shall not have any liability for any misrepresentation (express or implied) contained in, or for any omissions from, the information in this book. This disclaimer of liability applies to any damages or injury, whether based upon consumer law, negligence, or any other cause of action.

Foreword

I will never forget the moment I got the call … I was at work and the receptionist called out to me that my sister was on the phone.

I never expected the words I was about to hear.

I picked up the phone and Amanda said, 'I have MS.'

I literally fell to the floor.

I was devastated.

Watching my twin sister go through her first flare-up of MS was incredibly difficult, for many reasons. As a child I battled my own autoimmune disease, so I knew what was ahead of her.

All I could think about was how can I take it all on for her, so that she doesn't have to experience what was coming.

Watching Amanda go through her own experience of illness, I saw that we both battled a similar recovery. It was uncanny and incredibly difficult to watch, but it also opened my eyes to how this must have felt for my family watching me go through physical deterioration and recovery from a serious illness. The powerlessness that they must have felt. I felt this deeply for my sister.

I knew all I could do was just be there with her.

True to form, the extrovert that Amanda is took the battle head-on and focused her mindset on her own journey of recovery. And she did just that. With a lot of hard work and determination.

Amanda and I are just built that way ... when things get tough, we only see options on how to fix things. It becomes our only focus. Of course, we are human, and we pondered the what ifs and whatnots, but it doesn't take us long to get ourselves into a mindset that motivates us to become educated on all we could do to be better.

Amanda researched her disease extensively, and she found solutions that have helped her recover from a potentially devastating outcome.

Over time, through daily discipline and the hunger and drive to be better, she adopted these key principles in her daily life, and Amanda feels incredibly lucky and grateful to remain in full remission, whilst maintaining her health and mind protocols that she has now mastered.

I have learnt so much from Amanda, and I know that you will too by reading her experiences and what she has discovered that helped her recover from her own illness of multiple sclerosis.

For those who don't suffer from a serious illness, this book has the fundamental tools for anyone who wants to learn how to be a healthier and happier version of themselves, in all aspects of life.

One thing I have learnt is that when the student is ready, the teacher will come.

If this book resonates with you, then you are ready to learn some amazing principles and tools that will take your health and confidence to the next level, which will in turn give you empowerment and a sense of wellbeing – mentally, emotionally, and spiritually.

Our journeys are our own sacred paths ... Always remember: You are your own guru.

Nicole, Amanda's twin sister.

Contents

Testimonials	i
Disclaimer	ii
Foreword	iii
Introduction	1

Chapter 1
When Life Gives You Lemons — 7

Chapter 2
Flexibility Builds Resilience — 9
The importance of resilience — 14
My formula for resilience — 18
Flexibility promotes repair — 26

Chapter 3
Stress vs. Repair Pathways — 37
Stress and survival pathways — 39
Growth and repair pathways — 44
Autopilot vs. honeymoon states — 47

Chapter 4
What Causes Stress? — 55
A time of stress for me — 56
Barriers to wellness — 61
Barriers to overcoming stress — 65
What you can do about it — 69

Chapter 5
What We Believe Is What Matters — 73
Our beliefs have a big impact — 79
How you can believe — 83

Chapter 6
The Power of the Mind — 87
Learning to go within — 90
The link between pain and emotion — 94

Chapter 7
The Mind-Body Connection — 97
Identifying our beliefs by our reactions — 99
The reticular activating system — 103

Chapter 8
The Art of Bending Like Bamboo — 106
Bending with change — 108
Dealing with change — 110

My model of change	112
How I learned to Bend Like Bamboo	118
What is multiple sclerosis?	123

Chapter 9
The Power of Kinesiology	126
Qi Flow	130
Acupuncture studies	131

Chapter 10
The Bend Like Bamboo Program	135
The power of self-belief and resilience	136
Happy mind	142
Happy body	145
Happy food	152
Connection	158
Journaling and gratitude	164
Bend Like Bamboo for work, school and sports performance	168
How Bend Like Bamboo can help you	170

Chapter 11
Ideas vs. Beliefs	174
Align your goals with positive beliefs	174
My turning point	177

Chapter 12
The Pineapple Effect	179
You can change your mind	184
Follow your joy	188
A new me and a new career	203

Chapter 13
Reassessing Goals	210
A rebuild of my mind, body and life	212

About the Author	219
Appendix	221
Bend Like Bamboo and the anatomy of resilience	223
References	226
Acknowledgements	229

Introduction

In life we experience change every single day. Every now and then, life brings a bigger change that can feel like a setback – like divorce, illness, or a beginning or ending, professionally or on a personal level. With a flexible mindset we can perceive our rock-bottom moments as miracles and a redirection that is for our highest good. They can also be the very catalyst that propels us forward to daringly walk an unknown path, that is as scary as a black abyss.

How we respond to stress and change can impact on the choices we make, and the health of our minds and bodies. Our ability to rise above and be bigger than our setbacks can be the key to seeing our obstacles as opportunities to grow and become our fullest potential.

If we can see our setbacks as changes that happen in life, designed to set us onto a new path, then we can relax and adapt. I believe that what we go through in adversity teaches us valuable skills and lessons, assisting us to evolve and grow.

Our ability to acquire knowledge and to then integrate it into a new way of being in the world, can navigate us to understand the meaning of our lives, seeing our circumstances from a higher perspective. This requires us to learn how to live with a strong heart, a quiet mind, more patience and discipline. A difficult adventure at times, if we have not learned to adapt to change and are rigid from stress. We also cannot see these critical moments as opportunities that can changes our lives for the better.

When we are stressed, we can be rigid, less creative and less open to possibility. That is why I believe that flexibility builds resilience and building resilience in our mindset can improve our physical and emotional wellbeing.

That is how I came across the power of flexibility. On my own personal journey, recovering from illness or when I have had to heal from loss or grief, like many of us, I have had to rebuild my mind, body and life several times. When we are feeling exhausted, stressed or unmotivated, it can be difficult to apply a flexible mindset that can allow us to be more resilient and solution-focused. Learning how to master that art of flexibility can help us in this process, optimising our wellbeing, our ability to heal and an opportunity to learn and grow from life's adventures.

Our ability to develop an anchor within ourselves, reducing stress and shifting old beliefs, can radically change our health and the path of our lives. This process requires flexibility so that we can change our minds about 'the stories' we tell ourselves. It took me many years to understand this, and the importance of checking in with myself to reconcile the health of my thoughts and inner environment. If we get stuck and forget to do that, we can spend our entire life believing a redundant story that we have been telling ourselves, sometimes for a lifetime.

When stressed, we can revert to old programs that can lead us to believe that we are not good enough, smart enough, successful enough or lovable enough. Suppressing stuck anger, grief, shame or fear creates toxic energy that become stuck in our bodies. In the same way that off food can make us sick, toxic emotions also impact the health of our mindset, our moods, how we show up in our lives, and our ability to heal.

Introduction

We can become masters at suppressing difficult emotions and it becomes familiar to live our lives disconnected in this cycle of sabotage. This is stressful and living in this inner conflict can present as pain or inflammation in the body. When we sabotage our lives, this impacts our ability to make things happen for ourselves. When we are stressed and disconnected, we can find ourselves attracting toxic relationships, life feels like a struggle, and we end up using our precious energy engaged in unnecessary conflict, instead of using it to repair.

On my journey I realised there had to be a better way. I learned that untangling a lifetime of unhealthy patterns and rigidity, to transform the deepest subconscious parts of myself, required flexibility. With an elevated perspective and a more flexible mindset, we can see our world with fresh eyes and a higher understanding of our lives.

No matter what you have gone through in life, you can overcome it. Everything you are going through right now is designed to help you to grow and evolve. The aim is not to change what is going on externally. The question is, can you hold centre, can you train yourself to anchor deeper within amongst the change? Can you learn to bend like a bamboo tree? So that you can be flexible without snapping when the wind comes.

We can't escape the challenges that we will face; how we navigate them is what matters. That is how we build our resilience, self-belief and confidence, and this is how we can heal and grow. We can't go around them; we must go into and through them, facing our fears. Building and returning to an inner anchor that helps us to hold centre through life's ups and downs. Our ability to transform ourselves from the more difficult times that we face, requires us to lean into uncertainty and the unknown. This book explores how to do that with more trust and grace, amongst life's forces that are out of our control.

I stand here today against all odds. At age 24 I was diagnosed with multiple sclerosis (MS). At the age of 29, I was paralysed and was faced with never walking again. I discovered that a flexible mindset impacts everything that matters: our body's ability to repair, how happy and resilient we are, and our ability to reimagine what can be possible for our lives.

I wrote this book to share my story and the lessons I learned along the way when I had to learn how to walk again. Recovering from a debilitating illness, I researched theories and studied East and West concepts that I share in each chapter, with tips and actionable tools to help you to apply more flexibility in your life. I still use these tools every single day in a maintenance program, as they continue to be so useful. I will also share references in footnotes and resources in the Appendix at the end of the book.

I have been so lucky to experience a remission from MS that has remained consistent for over a decade. I have also seen incredible transformations at my private practice. Every time that I have the privilege to assist clients through their own journey of transformation, I am amazed by what can be achieved.

As a trained Sports Kinesiologist, I specialise in multiple sclerosis and autoimmune disease. I help my clients to destress and reset their minds, bodies and lives. As a resilience trainer, I help individuals to uncover blind spots, to achieve their personal and professional goals. How do I do this? I teach people how to Bend Like Bamboo.

I opened my private practice in 2014, after winning a Go for Gold Scholarship with MS Plus. Over the last decade I have worked with clients experiencing various symptoms and diseases. I am amazed by the power of our minds, the destruction and dysfunction we have the power to create within ourselves, and the healing that is also possible. I see clients in person and virtually on zoom,

I host retreats, deliver resilience and flexibility workshops to executives, kids and athletes. Bend Like Bamboo also has a blog, podcast and online program that can be found on my website and in the references at the back of this book.

This book is relevant for anyone who is on a journey to rebuild their mind, body and life. Perhaps you are feeling stressed, unmotivated, exhausted or unwell. Maybe you have been lacking self-belief and confidence within yourself. Or you have been experiencing digestive issues, physical pain, anxiety or depression. Perhaps you are seeking guidance on a pathway forward after change, after experiencing a break-up, death or grief in your life? If you are looking to heal from illness or burnout, or you are simply wanting to thrive and perform on top of your game, then this book was written for you.

In this book we will explore the power of flexibility, our body's ability to heal and repair, how to build more resilience within ourselves, within our relationships and how the power of flexibility can help you.

I also had to Bend Like Bamboo when I was grieving, when my Mum and my dog died suddenly, 4 months apart in 2021. This process has also been helpful when I have rebuilt myself after loss from the ending of chapters in my life. My ability to boost resilience and flexibility was also important when I have wanted to perform at my best at work or in any situation that required me to be solution-focused.

I turned 40 on 30 March 2020, just before we locked down in the COVID 19 pandemic. I shared this milestone birthday with my twin sister, Nicole. Writing this book and digitalising my work has been cathartic for me. I have had the opportunity to review the tools again, helping me build resilience and flexibility in new ways, applying what I have learned to adapt to immense global change.

My intention for this book is to inspire you to go on a journey within, to feel inspired to overcome any setback that are you faced with. To feel empowered to give your mind and body the best environment to be flexible, adaptable and open to change.

So, giddy up and let's get started! Take your own notes – I recommend post-it notes, so you can make action notes as you go. I'm so honoured to share my journey with you, and to be a little part of yours. x

Chapter 1

When Life Gives You Lemons

*Change is the only constant in life.
One's ability to adapt to those changes will determine
your success in life.*

Benjamin Franklin, statesman, scientist and diplomat

Pins and needles. No, not again. A few days later, I felt a familiar weakness in my left arm, hand and leg. My symptoms were back.

I was only 24 years old. I'd just found a career I loved, and I was good at it. I was motivated, driven and happy. Life was wonderful in every possible way. But now I was on my way to meet my neurologist to hear the results of another MRI. I was in my 'coping Amanda' mode. I pushed the flickering fear aside. Everything is fine, I told myself. The MRI will show nothing. I was trying to stay positive, but the truth is I was disconnecting, in complete denial about how frightened I really felt.

I sat in the simple office chair across the desk from the neurologist. Papers were spread out in front of him, and his kind eyes glanced down and back up at me as he asked a few questions about how I was feeling and what impact the symptoms were having. Then he paused. 'Amanda, I am so sorry. Your results show that you have multiple scars on your brain, which means we can now diagnosis you with multiple sclerosis. We can do a spinal lumbar puncture to confirm the results if you like, but in my opinion it is conclusive.'

He continued speaking and I tried to nod bravely, but his voice began to fade. 'You have multiple lesions on your brain, a few on the right side and one on your brain stem ...' Suddenly everything was moving in slow motion, as if the laws of gravity no longer applied. I could see him looking at me and I knew he was speaking, but all I could hear was the hollow thump of my blood pumping in my head. Tears ran down my cheeks, but I couldn't feel them. I was numb.

'Will I be able to have a family one day?' I asked, surprised by the breathless urgency of my question.

'Many people live to be well and have families.' He went on to explain that if my MS ended up being benign, there was a chance my condition would not progress. But it also might, and there was no telling which way it would go. I nodded again, but this time I didn't feel brave. I felt vulnerable and exposed, and I ran from his office into the next room where I cried harder than I've ever cried before.

Chapter 2
Flexibility Builds Resilience

Come to the edge, he said.
I am afraid, I said.
Come to the edge, he said.
I came, he pushed me, and I flew!

Christopher Logue, English poet

Flexibility in our mindset impacts on everything that matters: our body's ability to repair, how happy and resilient we are, and how we perform in times of setbacks.

In this chapter, we are going to explore:

- the incredible power of the brain and its connection to the body;
- tools to harness this power to promote growth and repair pathways; and
- moving from a place of just surviving to a place of thriving.

Our beliefs can cause inner conflict. Just wanting something is not enough to make it happen. That's because what we **believe** is what really matters, and this directly impacts on everything in our lives.

What we believe is connected to what we attract, the life we create and the health of our minds and bodies. For example, when we are stressed, we are focused on what we don't want, then fear builds up and we feel exhausted. This keeps us playing small in our lives, in a sabotage loop. When we are like this, we think from a rigid mindset that leads to more unhappiness and poor health.

There is a better way. We can train our brain to focus on what we do want, to feel positive and motivated, and to elevate our energy so we can notice more creative solutions around us.

Every second of every day, we have an opportunity to rewrite our story. We can choose how we will react, and we can change our minds about what is possible. You are the lead actor and director of your story, and you can write the script. When you start to see possibility within yourself, you start to see it everywhere.

No matter what I have been through – a rebuild of mind and body from illness, a reset after the ending of a relationship, or the grief of losing a loved one from death – I have learned that change is inevitable, and we experience change every day. Sometimes, life brings significant change that turns your world upside down, like divorce, death, a diagnosis, life events that force you to completely stop and reset. Such events force you to become a new version of yourself.

How we respond to change is a choice. When we can see challenging moments in our lives as opportunities, rather than obstacles, this opens us up to choose joy, healing and a transformation. When we can better manage our emotions, mood and reactions, we can make these moments a little more bearable. We can be more creative, happy and solution-focused.

In your life, I am sure that you have faced moments where you have felt like a part of you had to die, which were inevitably followed by a rebuild of mind, body and soul.

I have learned that flexibility builds resilience and building resilience allows us to not only maximise repair in our nervous systems, but also leads us on a path to reach our fullest potential. It can also give us the best environment to navigate change and the more difficult times that we face in life.

We all have a story; we have all been through and will continue to experience times of stress and change. Our ability to be flexible, and the concept of Bending Like Bamboo, is about the importance of who we are in those moments when we are faced with two paths. This becomes a moment of choice.

If we can practise flexibility in our minds, bodies and lives, we will be more adaptable and open to change when we are stressed, when we want to give up, or when we want to choose to give in. When we almost lose faith in ourselves and are painfully stretched out of our comfort zone. I believe that these are the moments that matter; who we are in these moments can change the trajectory of our lives.

I believe that flexibility builds strength, and a flexible mindset builds resilience. Bamboo is one of the most robust and flexible trees in the world, so flexible that globally, architects, builders and engineers are discovering new ways to harness the power of bamboo in the construction industry.

Bamboo is powerful, bamboo is flexible and bamboo is resilient. We can have those same qualities too and harness, apply and practise them in our everyday lives. A flexible attitude impacts everything that comes our way. Being open to change can have an enormous positive impact in our lives, professionally and personally.

To practise flexibility, it can be helpful to start the day with rituals that promote a quiet and calm mind, so that we can be more present in the moment. It is from this mindset we can change our minds about what we are believing, about our situation, then we can see things from different angles and from fresh perspectives. We can give new meaning to our circumstances and let go of whatever old story has become redundant for us. Any unresolved issues from the past can force us to relive an old story over and over again; welcome to what I call 'hell on earth'! Another word for this is pensiveness.[1]

Flexibility can help us to perform at our best. It fosters a connected and productive culture in the workplace and helps managers to be open to feedback and alter strategies accordingly. Flexibility helps leaders to lead with an elevated consciousness that radiates throughout the company's vision.

An analogy I frequently use with my clients, is to imagine you are standing on top of a mountain. When we are stressed it is like seeing life from the bottom of the mountain; all we can see is what is in front of us, a limited perspective. When we are stressed, we are not solution-focused, we are more reactive. It is from this limited perspective that we access lower dense emotions of anger, fear, worry, guilt and shame.

If we can push ourselves out of our comfort zone and shift our energy to support a more elevated mindset, we can promote more flexibility. In a morning meditation, you can imagine elevating to the top of a mountain. From this more elevated perspective, we are in the same body, in the same life, but we can see things very differently. From this elevated view, we can see all the streets, we can connect all the dots, we have a higher view and a greater understanding. It feels like things are happening for us, not to us. We can access more elevated emotions like joy, love, compassion, forgiveness and resilience.[2]

Resilience is our ability to step into the person we know we are ready to be, to create the life we really want. It is how

---

[1] - Definitions of pensiveness. Deep serious thoughtfulness. Overthinking, brooding, nostalgic hankering after the past, living in the past or future rather than in the present moment.

[2] - David Hawkins work on Letting Go - David R. Hawkins, M.D., Ph.D., is a nationally renowned psychiatrist, physician, researcher, spiritual teacher, lecturer, and speaker on the subjects of advanced spiritual states, consciousness research, and the realisation of the presence of God. He began working in psychiatry in 1952 and has published original research with Nobel Prize winners that helped revolutionise psychiatry.

we back ourselves when we are afraid. How we reset and ground ourselves when we feel overwhelmed, and how we support ourselves through change that is inevitable in our lives. It is how to feel safe and okay among the chaos. When we see life from a mountain top:

- we have a higher understanding, allowing us to connect the dots
- we are open to change and are more flexible
- we can see through other people's eyes and perspectives
- we can see betrayal, money blocks, poor health or sabotage with a fresh insight
- we can access a mindset that allows us to be more solution-focused
- we can be more present and kinder to ourselves and loved ones

The importance of resilience

What is resilience, and why is it so important? I believe that resilience is the ability to dig down deep when things get tough, when we want to give in, when the odds are stacked against us, or when life changes direction. In such times, our ability to manage stress directly relates to how successful, healthy and happy we are.

When we are resilient, we can transform a closed mindset into a growth one; we are better able to change our minds about how we feel, what we believe about ourselves, and what can be possible for us.

Resilience is not a gift; it is like a muscle that can develop from experience and training. It is a learned skill that we can all master. When faced with change, we can typically escape or elevate:

- We escape when we betray our inner voice and detach from guidance.

- We elevate when we overcome our obstacles and fears and there is lasting transformation.

I believe our reaction is dependent on how anchored we are within ourselves, and how solid our foundation is. I believe that resilience is also the ability to adapt and innovate; it is when pain strengthens us, allowing us to dig down deeper and realise our potential. It is our ability to push ourselves out of our comfort zone to grow. It is our ability to manage stress and change. It is the ability to face adversity head-on and push forward into unchartered territory. It is the ability to maintain balance, despite chaos or change in our environment; the ability to rebuild our lives and become our fullest potential. Resilience is the ability to discover our light within, and the ability to rewrite our old story and take responsibility for our reactions and choices.

No matter what I have been through in my life, my ability to be flexible has allowed me to be more resilient in the moments that mattered.

I have a resilience podcast, blog and YouTube channel called *Bend Like Bamboo*, where I interview special guests about what resilience means to them. I love to learn about other people's stories and how they have overcome adversity in their lives. On the podcast, I have the pleasure to meet and share some surprising and inspiring stories of resilience with special guests: men and women, leaders in business, celebrities, and some of the country's most loved and respected people. Together, we explore the topic of resilience, their story and what they have learned after overcoming some amazing things in their lives.

Many of the guests said that resilience is about our ability to push forward into uncertainty. Others said it is our ability to be vulnerable, kind and soft with ourselves, when we are stressed.

On the podcast, I have learned that resilience is how we show up for ourselves when we feel overwhelmed. How we anchor within ourselves helps us to regulate our emotions and our reactions, so that we can understand what they mean for us on a deeper level. With clarity and adaptability we can make better choices.

When we embody an anchor within, just as a bamboo tree is anchored in the soil, we can be more flexible. With a more adaptable mindset, we can shift our perspective to an elevated view. We know what people or circumstances to walk away from that are no longer good for us. We also have the courage to show up for ourselves when it is time to walk towards situations and opportunities that are important for our growth.

Take action
Relax and reconnect. To get you started, I recommend daily routines for your mind and body to boost connection and relaxation like meditation and journaling. When we feel safe we are more able to adapt to change.

What can you do daily to push yourself out of your comfort zone?

- ✓ Complete a task at the bottom of your to-do list.
- ✓ Add a wellness ritual into your day.

Laugh at yourself
Don't take life too seriously. Do less, have fun and enjoy the journey. Joy is part of the healing process. Show up and be fun, do the work and be reliable and accountable.

Allow your emotions to guide you
Practice getting out of your head, being as present as possible with an open heart. Your morning rituals will help you to capture this state. Can you maintain this state when you are stressed or challenged?

Exercise: The meaning of resilience
What does resilience mean to you? As a practical exercise …

- Think about what you experience internally, when stressed or going through change.
- Think about what you experience externally, when stressed or going through change.

- Think of an experience you have recently been through that stretched you.
- Think of the person you were before this event, who you are now, how you grew, and what you learnt as a result.

My formula for resilience

Anchor - Letting Go + Flexibility = Resilience
(A - LG + F = R)

Anchor

Your anchor is your foundation. A bamboo is anchored, is flexible, and can bend in direct proportion to the wind without breaking. Discovering your inner anchor is the end result of diving deeper within, building a rock-solid foundation.

In your own life, if you focus on flexibility, your experiences can give you the opportunity to master your own anchor. Your anchor is who you are, what you stand for, and knowing what you are made of. Once discovered, this realisation remains with you and will permeate into your relationships and how you show up in your life.

Think of it as a thermostat maintaining a consistent inner temperature, despite any change of weather on the outside. Can you practise maintaining a calm mind, a strong heart, feeling anchored in your body when the turbulence, change or perceived setbacks come?

This ability has a direct relationship with how happy we can be, within ourselves, our relationships, how well we can perform, the decisions that we make, and how we show up in the world. We can awaken to a sense of guidance that is accessed with a quiet mind, and the ability to sit with ourselves and our thoughts.

We can flow through life, knowing what to walk away from when it is not right for us. We know what opportunities to move towards, that align with our growth. We can observe our reactions and link them to shadows within ourselves that require light and healing.

Thermostat analogy

A thermostat is a device that automatically regulates temperature, or that activates another device when the temperature reaches a certain point. When we are stressed, confused, or overwhelmed, we forget to turn inward to utilise our inner resources, and we tend to search for answers externally. We deplete our energy reserves, and when we don't find what we are looking for, this can lead to more disappointment, stress and a lack of fulfilment.

The thermostat analogy helps us to connect to our inner anchor, despite inevitable change that happens in our life every day. It takes daily practice to build our inner thermostat. These daily rituals can help you in the more challenging times when they come. Starting and ending your day by returning to your inner anchor can make it easier to translate this practice into the course of your day, optimising a flexible and elevated mindset.

When we understand that we have the power to choose our reactions with a quiet mind and a strong heart, we can discover our unique superpowers. We will better understand what we are made of, knowing ourselves and what matters to us on a deeper level.

No matter what you are going through right now, believe that you can overcome it. You will believe it when you can learn how to back yourself and show yourself that you can regulate your inner thermostat.

When I've been faced with adversity and the darker times in my life, there was always a moment when I knew that I had a choice. I could either give up and stay the same, choosing the safe option. Or I could choose to change, to step up and answer my 'call to adventure'.[3] This is the very thing that makes us love the popular formula of the hero's journey by Joseph Campbell, which plays out in all the movies we love and watch repeatedly, such as *Alice in Wonderland*, *Star Wars*, *Karate Kid* and *Billy Elliot*.

To live life to your fullest potential, ask yourself: Am I listening to my call to adventure? How will I react when the going gets tough? That is what I call 'doing the work'! When no one is watching, how authentic are you really towards yourself?

You may be dissatisfied with life because of financial hardship, divorce, betrayal or illness. But these setbacks are the very catalysts that propel us to be the next version of ourselves we are ready to be. To a new path that awaits, and it is all part of our next stage of growth. These critical decisions move us from one world to another. Can you let go of old aspects of yourself that need to burn off, to let in the new?

> *You cannot discover new oceans, unless you have the courage to lose sight of the shore.*
>
> **André Gide, French author**

We discover our inner gold as we transcend the chaos, but friction is necessary. It is supposed to feel hard; you are meant to walk down paths that feel unpaved and unfamiliar. Waiting for you on your journey is your inner dragon that you must face and slay; the shadow aspects of yourself that you have the power to transform and heal.

---

[3] - The Call to Adventure sets the story rolling by disrupting the comfort of the Hero's Ordinary World, presenting a challenge or quest that must be undertaken. The Call throws the Ordinary World off-balance and establishes the stakes involved, if the challenge is rejected.

There is always a choice, and you get to choose how you will respond. Crisis encapsulates danger and opportunity, and the reality is that we are full of potential. The question begs: Can you go beyond your limits of perceived possibility? It's not how we fall but how we rise again that matters.

Exercise: Finding your anchor

Ask yourself:

- When do you feel anchored?
- What are your daily rituals?
- What is different about you and your day when you start it anchored within?
- What change do you notice in your reactions? In your performance and decision-making skills?

My go-to pillars of health help me to focus on developing my inner anchor daily:

- ✓ Mind – journal
- ✓ Body – movement
- ✓ Food – hydration, nutrition
- ✓ Connection – inner anchor, meditation, connection to relationships

Minus, letting go

Becoming a master at letting go requires the release of redundant beliefs and stories that are not aligned with our highest good, our fullest potential and what we are truly capable of.

We can identify and let go of our attachments, the monkey mind, disempowering words, thoughts, feelings and beliefs. Most importantly, we can let go of the stories we tell ourselves, that keep us suffering in a state of sabotage.

Our ability to manage stress is directly related to the amount of suppressed and repressed feelings we have accumulated. The more emotional pressure we can surrender and let go, the less vulnerable we are to the stress response and stress-related illnesses.[4]

Letting go is the ability to question our thoughts and stories, to differentiate between a victim state of blame, to acknowledge how our setbacks have served us, which then allows us to grow and capture the lessons.

Letting go allows us to let things come and go in our life naturally, without grasping, as we move forward into the unfamiliar. This can help us to experience more in life and this developing courage fulfils us. Letting go is the ability to let go of judgement, being the observer in our lives, separating the unnecessary dialogue from the necessary.

Mastering the art of letting go leads us to a path of receiving joy, love and an ability to manifest our desires. It leads us to think positively, receiving more joy in our daily life, rather than getting stuck in the habit of worry and assuming worst-case scenarios.

Exercise: Mastering the art of letting go

Ask yourself:

- Are you good at letting go?
- What old stories or beliefs do you think about from the past that limit you now?

---

[4] - *Letting Go* by David Hawkins. David R. Hawkins, M.D., Ph.D. is a nationally renowned psychiatrist, physician, researcher, spiritual teacher, lecturer and speaker about advanced spiritual states, consciousness research, and the realisation of the presence of God. He began working in psychiatry in 1952 and has published original research with Nobel Prize winners that helped revolutionise psychiatry.

- When you have let something go that has not served you, what did you notice?
- What change do you notice in your reactions?
- What change do you notice in your performance and decision-making skills?

Case study

I worked with a girl who wanted to thrive in her sales role but had a fear of the sales calls and execution. We dove deeper to realise that it was her fear of being criticised that led to a lack of confidence, which impacted on her performance. It was an old story that she had not let go of, that no longer aligned with what she wanted to create in her life.

Creating a flexible mindset and bringing this into her awareness allowed her to create a new story. Creating new thoughts, emotions and actions helped her to rewire her brain to adapt and change.

Thinking moved to feeling, then to being, acquiring knowledge and embodying this into a way of being. Now she is winning awards for the leads that she makes from her sales calls.

Plus, flexibility

Flexibility in our mindset impacts on everything that matters: our body's ability to repair, how happy and resilient we are, and how connected we feel. Flexibility in our mindset allows us to change our minds about old stories and beliefs that conflict with our goals and what we are wanting.

Flexibility in our body mirrors a flexible mindset; this can be optimised with a movement and stretch program.

Flexibility in our soul feels expansive when we are aligned, walking our talk, living a life of meaning, higher understanding and purpose. When the soul stops growing, you can feel it deep within. Could it be possible that our bodies try to communicate to us through ailments, symptoms and disease? Can you listen more closely to your inner guidance and intuition in your daily anchoring practice?

When we are flexible, we can choose our thoughts, we can ask more questions and react more consciously. We no longer need to be right all the time and can see from many more perspectives. We can let go of inner resistance and accept what is, rather than needing things to be different. Some questions for you to think about …

- What do you need to let go of?
- How can you be more flexible?
- What is your old story that you find yourself stuck in when you are stressed?
- Can you reimagine what can be possible for you, if you let go of your old story?
- What would you wear, how would you walk, how would you talk?
- Can you visualise a new version of yourself that can become this new reality?

Flexible vs. inflexible mindset

There are many benefits of mastering a flexible mindset:

- ✓ We are more joyful.
- ✓ We are more adaptable to change.
- ✓ We prioritise a happier life.
- ✓ We are more resilient.
- ✓ We can see more possibilities.
- ✓ We can see obstacles as opportunities.

- ✓ We are kinder and more connected.
- ✓ We promote repair in the mind and the body.
- ✓ We have a competitive edge.

Here are some of the issues we can face with an inflexible mindset:

- ✗ inflammation and disease
- ✗ a compromised immune system
- ✗ pain in the body
- ✗ self-sabotage behaviour
- ✗ disengagement at work, at home and within our relationships
- ✗ lack of joy, stuck in a punishment cycle
- ✗ biochemically: issues with digestion, hormones and energy
- ✗ emotionally: anxiety, inner criticism, suppression of our difficult emotions

Exercise: Embracing flexibility

Ask yourself:

- Are you good at being adaptable and flexible?
- When did you last have to adapt in your life?

Think of examples of when you have been more flexible in the past.

- What change did you notice in your reactions?
- In your performance and decision-making skills?

Flexibility promotes repair

When we are tired, stressed and anxious, we tend to overthink the future. We can become stuck in the past, living on autopilot. This impacts on our ability to be at our best, at home, at work and within our relationships. It is a mindset, and when we are stressed, tired and disengaged, we can believe there is no way out.

The truth is, we have no idea how adaptable we are. With a flexible mindset, we can change our minds about the stories we tell ourselves, we can find our inner anchor within ourselves. Expressing our lives from an inner thermostat that remains consistent can provide the emotional security and assurance that we seek externally, from within. When anchored, we are flexible, adaptable, and can reimagine what is possible in our minds, bodies and lives.

My twin's illness with Crohn's Disease

I'd now love to take you back to when I was a little girl. As a young girl, I was always on a mission to succeed; to experience and discover as much as I could, as quickly as I could. I was always inquisitive. The underlying theme in all that I searched for was to discover my 'why' and the meaning of life. In my teens, 20s and 30s, I had something to prove and I was itching to achieve it.

I am an identical twin and my grandmother 'Muma' moved in when Nicole and I were born. Mum didn't realise she was having twins (what the?) until late in the pregnancy (her gynaecologist had been away on holidays). Muma came over for a weekend to help and she stayed with us until the day she died, just twelve years ago in 2011. We were so lucky to effectively have two mums, and always felt very loved.

Our mother and grandmother were both born in Croatia, lived in France from 1956, then found solitude in Australia in 1960. Mum was about 25 years old when she met Dad and was working as a secretary at the time. She had been a model from age 19–22, and often spoke about her travels to Sydney and New Zealand with fondness and a gleam in her eye.

Nicole and I visited Croatia together in 2019 and met our aunty Zdenka and cousin Marko, who happens to be the same age as us. It was an experience I will never forget. We reunited after last seeing them when they visited Australia 32 years ago. We are so grateful we got to see them before the travel restrictions started in 2020. We now keep in regular contact on WhatsApp.

Dad was an entrepreneur at heart and had enormous passion for his work. He worked long hours and travelled a lot. I have wonderful memories of us all skiing together at Mount Buller. Although the time we spent together was limited, I am grateful for the education and opportunities that he provided for us. I think I found his absence difficult as a child; I really missed him being a part of important family moments. As an adult, I have learned that he did his best at the time and loved us in his own way.

In Dad's older years, we have connected much more, which I love. We have been able to chat about his perspective and his choices. As an adult, it's been very healing for me to see things through his eyes. This communication has enabled me to let go and shift some of the ideas I had created about my value and worth, when he was unavailable to spend time with us as a family.

Thanks to Val (our Nana on Dad's side), a violinist in the Melbourne Symphony Orchestra, we started playing instruments at a young age. Nicole and I developed a passion for music, playing the flute, piano and violin, as well as training in classical singing at our school, Presbyterian Ladies College (PLC).

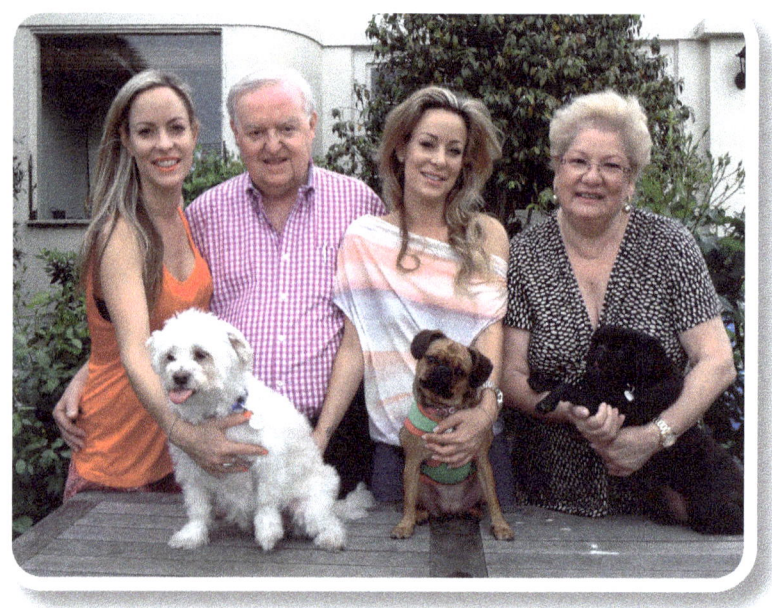

Amanda, Noel (Dad) Nicole (Sister), Lisa (Mum), Billy, Chloe and Henry

When we were 11 years old, life took a turn. My twin sister, Nicole, was diagnosed with Crohn's disease. She was in constant pain, one of the worst cases seen back then in 1991. I have memories of her rocking backward and forward, doubled in pain, Mum and Muma comforting her with cold face washers.

The medications caused difficult side effects for Nicole, making it so much worse. As a side effect of her medications, and probably as an extension of her condition, Nicole developed Rheumatoid arthritis. She started losing an immense amount of weight and at her worst weighed just 19 kilograms. It was awful seeing someone I loved so deeply go through such a hard time.

Nicole grew extra hair on her body and had massive amounts of fluid retention around her face and stomach, due to high doses of prednisolone. Her growth was stunted for a few years. As she declined in health, we didn't look as alike anymore; I went on to grow into a teenage body with boobs and braces.

We were 6 weeks premature when we were born on 30 March 1980. The hospital put us in separate humidicribs, and I believe this early experience of separation exacerbated when Nicole and I were apart while she was unwell. Abandonment was already an open wound and led to a lot of grief and resentment for both of us to work through as we grew up.

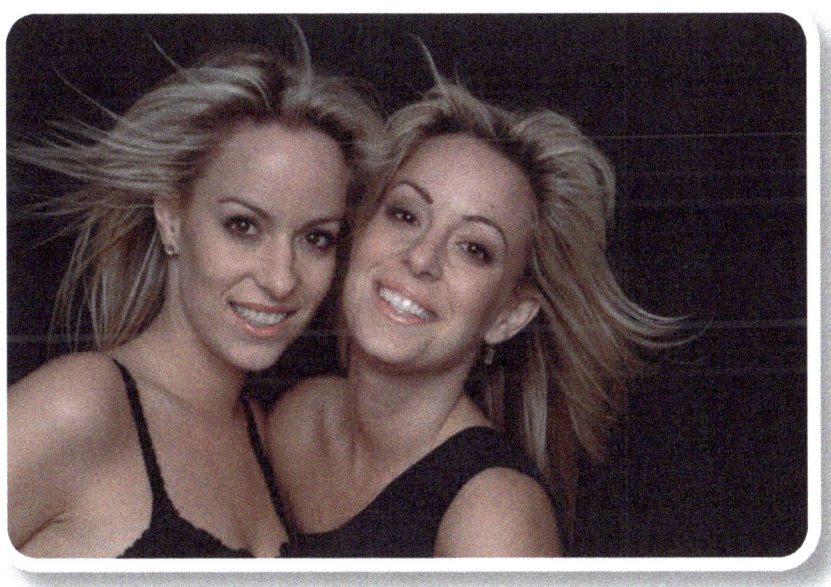

Amanda & Nicole's album cover

Our twin connection is real; we both felt 'twin pains' at that time and I remember feeling them at school. My connection to Nicole is always strong, even when we are apart. There is nothing I can really compare it to; I think it feels different to the connection of a sibling, and different to the love and connection you feel with a soul mate. Nicole and I have a half-sister, Claire, who Dad had with his ex-wife before he met Mum. We'd all spend time as a blended family for dinners growing up. Claire has two kids, Chester and Poppy my niece and nephew.

Being a twin is a gift; you are aware that the unique connection you have with each other is truly profound. We finish each other's sentences, yet our personalities are so different we can drive each other up the wall! Our fights can be epic, but they are short and never last more than a few days.

Whenever Nicole took a turn, there was a sudden overwhelming sense of doom in my belly, followed by a teacher coming into my classroom to get me to the hospital. Nicole had to spend weeks at a time in The Royal Children's Hospital when she had a flare-up, and I was usually by her side, sitting next to her hospital bed. However, I had no control over having to go to school and I hated going without her. She was my BFF and we hated being apart.

But as twins we lost our innocent bond – not just because we didn't look the same anymore, but because we went from experiencing life together to being separated a lot of the time. Even when Nicole was home, she wasn't well enough to spend time with anyone; she was mainly in bed, in Mum's or Muma's arms, just trying to survive the pain and her illness.

To this day, all that separation still haunts and affects us, as we learn to reshape our story and what we believed about ourselves, our situation, and the damage that requires healing after an illness changes a family. This trauma affected how much love we were able to give and receive from one another in our adult years. But we have worked on it and have done a lot of therapy, both solo and together.

Growing up, I missed our connection deeply. So when we disconnect today, it is a massive trigger for me. We continue to learn how to shift our pain to heal our wounds, so that we can be grateful and happy again.

Being an extrovert, I made more friends at school … I had to. I saw my school counsellor regularly and found it incredibly helpful to learn how to reach out and communicate. This is a skill that has served me later in all the careers I've had as a personal assistant, as a performer and now as a Kinesiologist and as a speaker. Nicole, more of an introvert, internalised a lot of her loneliness and pain. I desperately wanted to be next to her in the hospital, but I had to go to school. I fought to be there with her, but I was too young and didn't want to make a difficult situation any worse. I learnt how to navigate the world without her. I had to become a new version of myself, adopting new routines so I could exist in a world without my twin and other half.

Nicole's illness made me question my own mortality, and I had to contemplate what my life would be like if I lost her. As a twin, I was also warned that, statistically, I could get as sick as Nicole. I also missed my mother; she was so stressed and drained from everything she and Nicole were going through, there wasn't much time or energy left to connect with me. This led to me forming beliefs that I was not supported or worthy of love and protection. When our needs aren't met as children, we can become angry and resentful, something I have had to work through over the years to acknowledge, process and heal. It is important to see our situation with fresh eyes as we get older, as our parents are also humans and are dealing with difficult times in their lives. I know that for many years, holding onto my anger also stopped me from forgiving, moving forward and receiving all the love my mum wanted to give me in my life. We made peace with this on the last day she had on earth, a very difficult lesson I took with me after she passed away to not wait so long. But I am so glad Nicole had Mum by her side through the hardest time of her life. Mum was such an amazing carer, something I would admire and witness again as I watched her love and care for Muma full time at home, at the end of her life. Muma, our grandmother, passed away 6 August 2011 at age 86. We loved her so much; she was a second mother to Nicole and I. We were so blessed.

I felt helpless and I didn't know how to make my twin feel better. As a kid, I was trying to piece together the chaos of home. Everyone became so stressed; it was hard on us all. Nicole flatlined and nearly died in hospital, twice. She remembers surrendering and giving in to the pain. I guess she'd had enough of being in constant pain, and her body just couldn't fight anymore. From Year 7 to the end of Year 9 she didn't go to school.

Unfortunately, Mum and Dad's marriage didn't survive. They grew apart for many reasons, something I would only come to understand as an adult. My family separated when I was 14 and in Year 9. Nicole was at her worst that year; we were all in survival mode, living in a constantly alarmed state, wondering if Nicole was going to make it through.

That same year, I had to leave PLC, due to financial difficulties, along with all my friends and secure network. I loved that school, particularly the arts; we'd spent half the time in the music school, singing and writing our own music together. After the end of Year 8, I went to Wesley College in Prahran, a co-ed school that was more formal than I had been used to. I initially struggled as I missed my support – not only at home, but at school as well. I was coping up to this point. On reflection, this was the critical point in my life when I began to unravel.

Nicole and Mum went to London for 6 weeks, to try a new treatment to save Nicole's life. That was a pivotal time in my life. I believe it was the year something switched inside me. I missed Mum and Nicole and had changed schools. It all became overwhelming; I could feel myself becoming a harder version of myself. I became angry and shut down. It was the longest time I was away from both Mum and Nicole, and it absolutely sucked. Thankfully, Muma was home with me running the house, and Dad would come home after work, but he was never emotionally available. He was stressed too, he began to take it out on me. His own father was unwell at the time, so Dad was juggling work, going to the hospital with Nicole at nights – I can't imagine the pressure. But I felt totally alone, in a very uncertain world.

A few months after Mum and Nicole got home, Grandad passed away. Most of the time I was in my room by myself feeling empty, scared, alone and uncertain about when there would be any relief, and wondering what would be around the next corner. I got used to feeling out of control. I lost the innocence I used to have when I could trust that all was safe, when I could go with the flow. I was on alert for the next thing to blow up. This is how I learned how to disconnect from my mind and my body, and I did it very well.

Our family learned to live this way, fearing the worst-case scenario. You could feel the joy being squeezed out of us. It really affected our mindset, how we treated each other, and how we felt within ourselves. It was difficult to stay connected as a family, through such a hard time.

Luckily, Nicole pulled through by the age of 17. The treatment in London worked, a combination of chemotherapy and a high dose of antibiotics treating tuberculosis. It worked so well she got off the steroids and all the drugs that were giving her such debilitating symptoms (often worse than the disease).

This does not mean I advocate against drugs or Western medicine; they can be highly effective and essential. Mark my words, if I am in an accident, if I have a diverticulitis flare-up (something I have experienced twice and will never forget), or if break my leg, I want you to take me to a surgeon. Particularly for acute trauma. In saying that, I have found that a wholistic and Eastern approach has managed to get to the bottom of health issues and MS symptoms I have had, in ways a drug was unable to. In my experience, I find an integrated and balanced approach works best for issues that have been brewing for long periods of time and that are stress-related.

Events, interactions and changes will come into our lives that will be stressful at times. When our nervous system perceives threat, it is not always from obvious things or events like an accident, running from danger, or finding ourselves frozen and in a stress response from the trauma of an accident.

I have learned that it can also feel like a matter of life or death when we become stressed from interactions within our relationships, a perceived lack of belonging, or a lack of connection within our families, which often leads to a disconnect within ourselves (I will go into more of this in the next chapter).

Our thinking, emotions and beliefs are connected to the biochemistry we fire from our brain, out into the system of our bodies. If we simplify this into two predominant pathways, one keeps us alive (the stress response) and one promotes rest, growth and repair. Could our thinking and emotions shift us into a survival state? If so, could we prioritise repair and healing from our thinking and beliefs? I went on a mission to research recovery and found that the answer to this question was 'yes'.

When we are in a stress response, it feels like we are disconnected, disengaged and even withdrawn. We can overthink, overanalyse and get stuck in our intellect, instead of our intuition. We burn glucose for fuel so that we can escape danger faster, and this can lead to weight gain, inflammation and a lack of wellbeing in the mind and body.

The opposite happens when we feel more connected, joyful and present. We are more engaged, creative and solution-focused. Feeling less stressed and more joyful, we can burn fat for fuel instead of glucose, which can promote weight loss and repair in our minds and bodies. This is the best environment we can give ourselves to navigate change, and to manage stress in our lives.

On my journey, this helped me to understand the difference between the sensations and the connected biochemistry of a more flexible and relaxed state that can promote repair vs. a stressed one that can lead to inflammation and degeneration. In my own experience living with MS, I knew I had to learn how to maximise growth and repair pathways and this is why it became my mission to not only learn how, but to integrate this knowledge into a new way of being in the world.

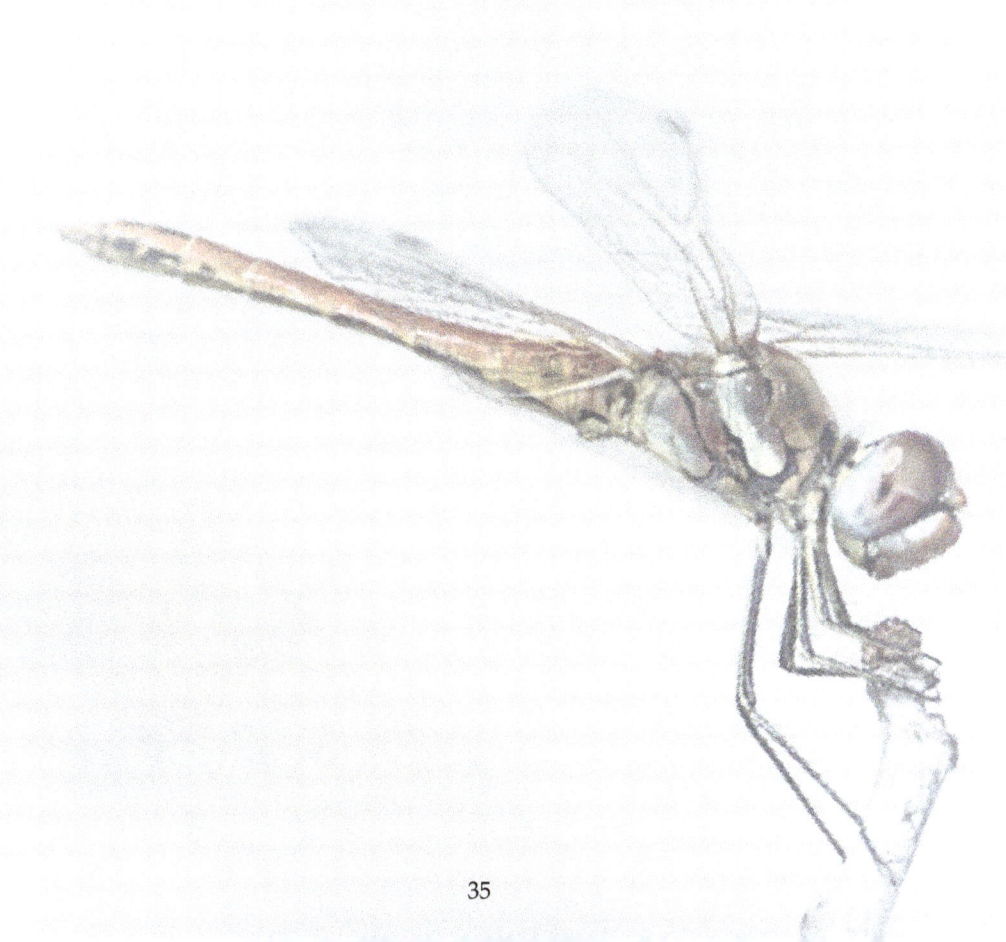

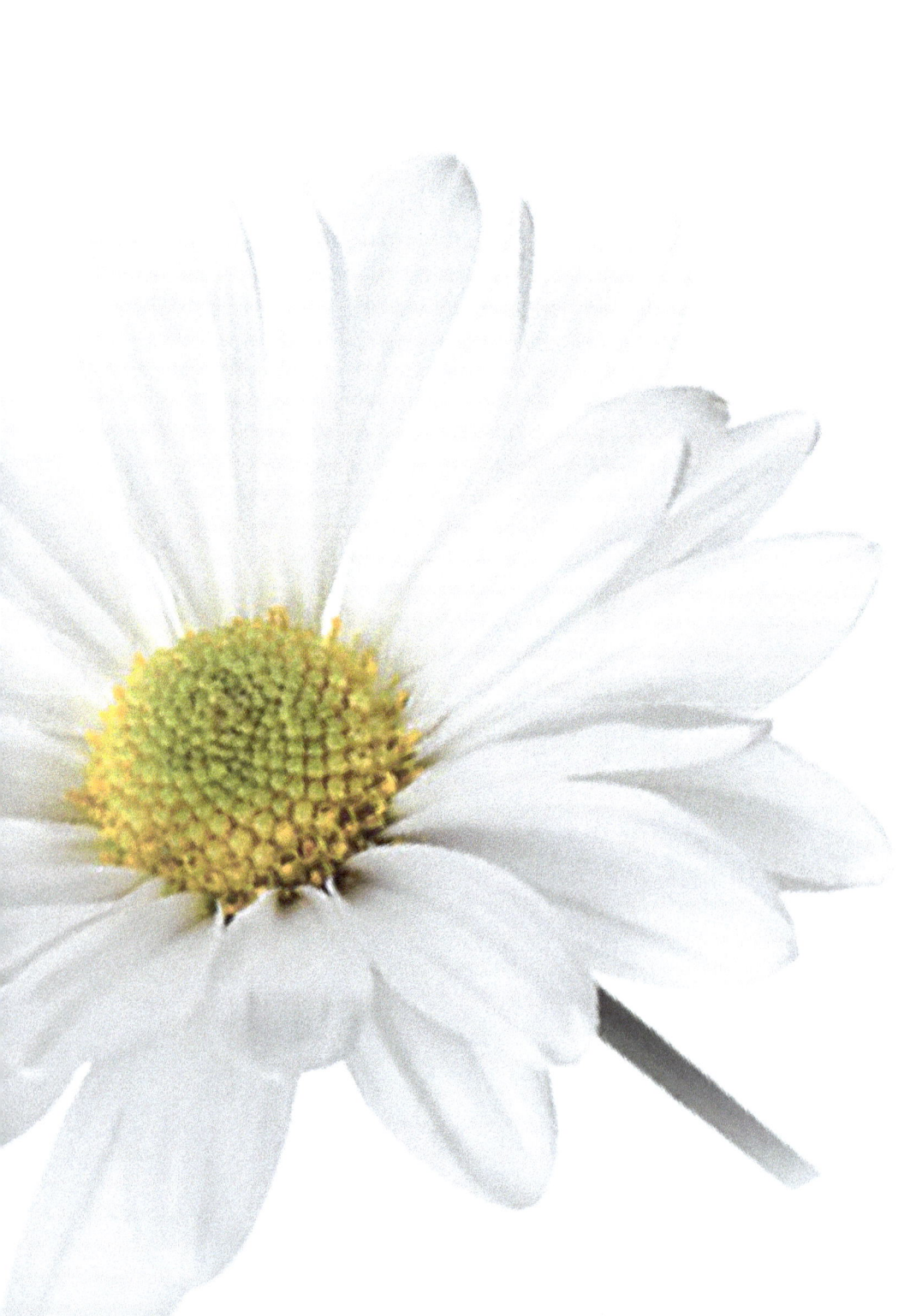

Chapter 3
Stress vs. Repair Pathways

In this chapter, we will explore the two pathways that we can fire in the body: stress and survival vs. growth and repair. If you are interested to learn more about the science behind these two pathways, I recommend researching Bruce Lipton's work, *The Biology of Belief*[5] and Joe Dispenzia's work.[6]

What we believe is what matters. When we continuously operate in a negative and stressed mindset, our immune system can become compromised, we can experience a loss in motivation and vitality, and our health may deteriorate. Not the best environment to optimise resilience. It is significant how much energy we can spend fearing worst-case scenarios, failure, not believing in ourselves or what could be possible for us.

Actions that mirror a negative mindset are often linked to low energy and procrastination, ramifications from long-term stress, or sometimes just feeling 'beige' about life. Believe it or not, disengaging from your life and living in a disconnected state drains a lot of energy, because it becomes an inner conflict and is not our most optimal state of being. It can be a way to protect ourselves from failure, an excellent way to sabotage.

I believe that our health is a mirror image of what we believe about ourselves and our circumstances. When we are faced with adversity, we become stressed and stretched, mentally and physically. When we are out of our comfort

---

5 - https://www.brucelipton.com/books/biology-of-belief
6 - https://drjoedispenza.com/

zone it can be stressful, and our nervous system can believe that it needs to protect us from perceived danger. After my recovery and thanks to the study of kinesiology and the work I do with my clients, I have become intrigued by the pattern of the two pathways we typically fire in the body: stress and survival vs. growth and repair.

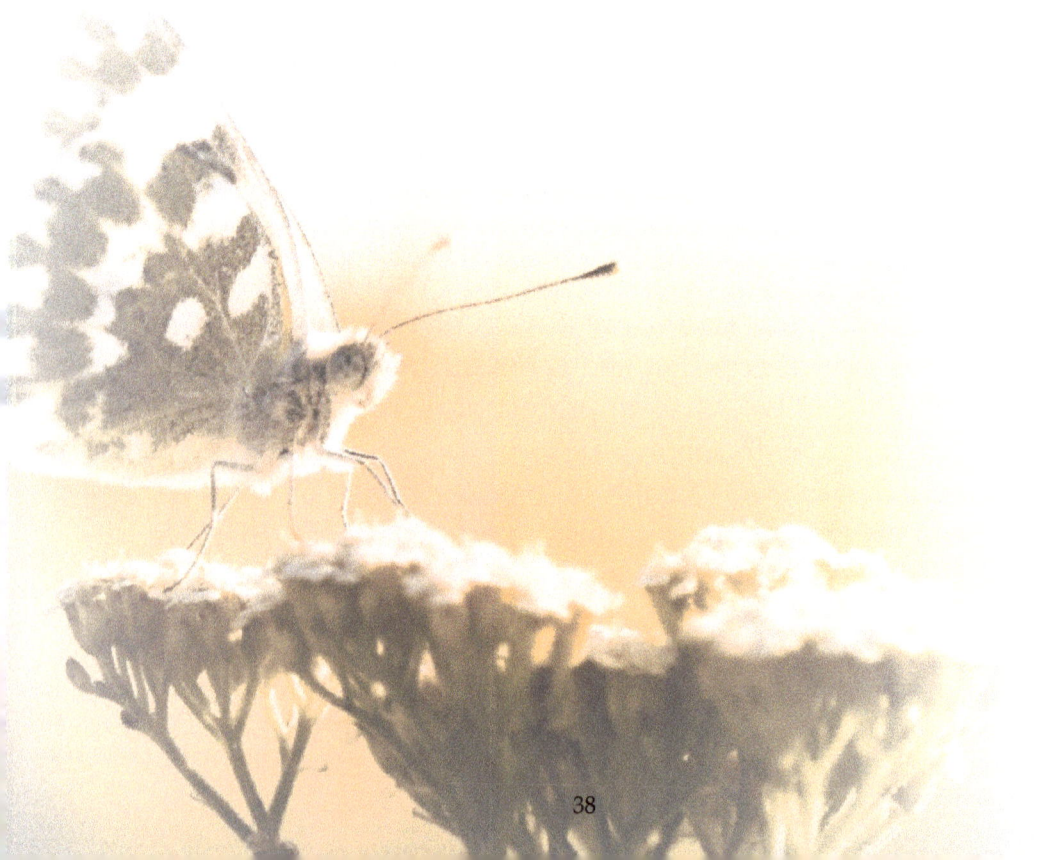

Stress and survival pathways

Survival mode occurs when our body believes it needs to keep us alive, so it goes into a fight, flight or freeze response. Switching 'on' was very useful back in the days when a man or woman had to run from a predator like a tiger. After escaping the danger, we would then turn 'off', relaxing back into a balanced state.

In our modern lives, our bodies can experience high levels of stress from problems like financial worries, family issues, difficult relationships or overworking to live up to someone else's expectations. As a result, an alarmed state can remain switched 'on' for long periods of time. Add to this the external stimulation from our addiction to digital media and you have a perfect storm for anxiety, disconnection, stress, inflammation and disease.

Our brain switches from survival mode into growth mode when our body believes or perceives that it no longer needs to protect us. When we are calmer, happier and not perceiving threat anymore, we can prioritise new pathways of growth and repair.

In Bruce Lipton's groundbreaking work, *The Biology of Belief* [7], he explains the ramifications of stress and the destructive pathway it leads to. This discovery was a game changer for my mind, body and life. I think it is so important to consistently question how we are, our thinking, how we feel, and what we believe.

---

7 - https://www.brucelipton.com

Feeling less stressed, we can be more present, adaptable and healthier human beings.

We are either firing in growth or survival mode, depending on how we interpret stress and our environment. Receptors around our cells consistently monitor our internal chatter and external environment, deciding how to respond and what signals to fire out to our body.

The brain's priority is to survive. A survival response will always take precedence, which means that when we are stressed, the safest way the brain knows to mitigate the risk is to process old memories, focusing on negative or worst-case scenarios.

Have you noticed that when you are stressed, you make decisions that keep you within your comfort zone? You may stick to the familiar when you feel frightened; for some of us, what is familiar can unfortunately be a survival program of 'I can't', 'That will never happen' or 'I am not good enough'.

Exercise: *Getting out of our comfort zone*

Ask yourself these questions:

- Is it familiar for you to feel inspired, alive and motivated?
- Do you intentionally try to get out of your comfort zone?
- Or has it become familiar to feel stuck in fear, lacking willpower and belief in yourself?
- Does your environment mirror what you want for yourself?
- Is there a conflict or resistance (your beliefs not aligning with your goals)?
- Are you thinking or believing that nothing is going right for you?

In an stressed state of fear, it can become familiar to stay small, to block enjoyment, to live in a punishment cycle, to feel unwell or exhausted. When in survival mode, there is a lack of integration between our intellectual, intuitive and emotional brain, and this can result in poor mental and physical health, inevitably leading to a lack of innovation and creativity. This is not an ideal environment to repair or thrive in; it undermines many areas of our lives, especially in the workplace where we spend so much of our time.

Four key types of stress

In my private practice, I address four key types of stress:

- physical (injuries, accidents, pain, traumas)
- emotional and mental (anxiety, depression, sabotage reactions)
- biochemical (toxins, nutrition, infection, pathogenic organisms like bacteria and viruses)
- environment and connection (relationships, finances, career, mind-reality conflict)

If we don't take time to notice when stress is affecting us and improve our state, we can get stuck in a rut of overthinking and worry. Fear can lead us to express cautious behaviour that lacks trust and inhibits our ability to think of creative solutions or possibilities. I have been through times when I have stopped following my gut feelings or intuition; I also see this cycle every day in my practice.

The good news is that it is possible to change how we perceive stress and our reactions to it. To relax and feel safe again, we need to be malleable and flexible, so we can be open to change and our perception of things. It is like our body needs to relearn how to turn 'off' into rest and repair and into balance, which involves rewiring the brain and the stories that we tell ourselves. This is a pathway to form new habits, thoughts and a new way of life.

My work has led me to discover the emotional links between physical stress and diseases. Linking our mental health and emotions with physical and biochemical imbalances, I believe, is key to optimising wellness and a happier life. It can be a path to optimal performance and a deeper connection in our lives. Unlocking this can be the best gift you ever give to yourself, shifting blocks you may have had for a long time, for the long haul.

In everyday life, I believe that we simply don't question our outdated thoughts and tightly held beliefs enough and doing so is pivotal for recovery. Imagine if we learned skills like this at school: believing in ourselves, resilience and kindness, managing stress as well as emotions and reactions. I wish I'd learned these skills growing up! I would have been able to understand myself and how to manage my stress levels much better, and it would have prevented so much suffering.

But I also now understand that the suffering and harder times in my life were required for me to learn. It is the actual act of going through the hard times, especially the parts I didn't believe I could overcome, that helped me to change my mind about what I was capable of, and what could be possible for me. That is how we reach our fullest potential, leading us to feel happier, wiser, healthier and stronger people. It is as if all our setbacks are purpose-built stages in the game of life, helping us move to the next stage of growth.

These tools have not only helped me to repair but have also helped to maximise my wellbeing in ways I never imagined possible. Learning the emotional links to my brain and nervous system, that had caused me stress, helped to calm down my nervous system and the neurological disease that literally paralysed me. It was like turning off the tap at the source. For me, it was a game changer.

If the body is stuck in a survival pattern, unable to turn 'off', it can be a reaction to current stress. But current stress can be triggering old unresolved issues we may not have fully processed or dealt with. I believe that stress, alongside a poor diet, unprocessed difficult emotions, a lack of self-love, and a perceived threat in one's environment are the perfect inflammatory storm, that can also lead to feeling disconnected, lacking in purpose, hope and direction.

Our unresolved mental and emotional stresses often manifest as physical symptoms, which are feedback and an invitation to look at what we are avoiding in our life. At Bend Like Bamboo, my clients who are going through this tend to present with glassy eyes, as though no one is home; their essence (spirit) appears absent from the body. A loss of brain integration and confusion can be observed as well, and a lack of mind-heart connection, which can present as anxiety and heart palpitations.

Growth and repair pathways

When our body is in a state of growth and repair, it is like activating the brakes in our parasympathetic nervous system. You know that feeling when you are on holiday, and you can really switch off? The body receives a signal from the brain to prioritise rest and repair, instead of survival. You may feel present and calm – people may even notice a sparkle in your eye! This energy is contagious and inspiring, because we are reconnecting back to ourselves and back out to the people in our lives. When you notice this in another person, it makes you feel connected too, and you can't help but subtly smile to yourself.

If we focus on being responsible for creating a life filled with joy, health and building a deeper connection within, this is also an optimal way to ripple kindness, compassion and love into others and out into our world. When we are in this state, we can heal, we can see our life from a higher perspective, we are more creative and solution-focused.

We can achieve our goals much faster when our body finds a better balance between the two pathways of survival and growth. So how do we learn how to balance our autonomic nervous system?[8]

Our mind and body are more malleable and suggestible to change when we are feeling good. When we feel safe, calm and joyful, we can let go of the past. We are kinder

---

8 - The parts of the nervous system (sympathetic and parasympathetic) that control muscles of internal organs (such as the heart, blood vessels, lungs, stomach and intestines) and glands (such as salivary glands and sweat glands).

and able to see situations from other people's eyes with compassion. Enthusiasm and hope are more accessible, and we can begin to change our minds about what is possible for us.

My four pillars of health

How can we begin to change our minds about what can be possible? What helps me are my 4 pillars of health: mind, body, food and connection.

Mind: You wash your body every day, but how do you wash your mind of the old story? The thoughts that you overthink in your head? You know that voice that holds you back, that makes you feel like you are not enough – the monkey mind, the fear, the doubt.

Body: Move your body every day, with stretches and exercises that are right for you. If you are not very mobile due to disability, get help from a specialist to find a way to move your body with therapies or stretching.

Food: When we eat better, we feel better. When we feel better, we are more adaptable, flexible, creative and solution-focused. We can promote more repair in the mind and body.

Connection: Reconnect back to yourself every day, especially when you are stressed. I do this with daily meditation in the morning and evening. Throughout the day, I try to take moments of presence to ground and anchor me back into my body.

Every month after my kinesiology session, I am working on something within myself. For example, I may be focused on bringing in more playfulness and joy, or slowing down, or letting go of an emotion of anger or shame. I like to write an affirmation on my bathroom mirror with a whiteboard texta, to help me think and feel in a new way, as I integrate this knowledge into a new way of being in my life. Shifting the biochemistry to promote growth and repair, instead of stress and survival.

> *Every day, in every way, I am getting better and better.*
> **Emile Coué, French psychologist**

This is my special mantra. What mantras do you say daily? Your inner dialogue is either helping you to elevate your mindset or is lowering it. Mantras can help to remind you to focus on your intention and your 'why'.

Autopilot vs. honeymoon states

It can be helpful to identify the difference between feeling stressed, and how it feels when you are calmer and more present. When we are stressed, it can feel like you have checked out, you feel disengaged.

The autopilot state (the unconscious)[9]

Because the subconscious brain is a million times more powerful than the conscious part of our brain[10], we rely on it when we are stressed. Our subconscious is where our beliefs, programs and habits are stored, and it's the part of the brain you use to function when you are in survival mode. Many people now live in this survival state for 95% of each day without realising it.

Our subconscious is our autopilot mode and is also the more powerful part of the brain. When we are tired, stressed or are perceiving threat, we divert to the more dominant programs of the subconscious. How many times have you driven home and, once there, realise you have no recollection of the streets you turned down or how you got there? That is because the subconscious is so powerful, it can manage the navigation, the motions needed to drive the car, and keep an eye on traffic while you are talking to your passengers and thinking about your to-do list, all at the same time!

---

9 - In "Mindfulness-Based Cognitive Therapy," Crane explains that "the term 'automatic pilot' describes a state of mind in which one acts without conscious intention or awareness of present-moment sensory perception.

10 - https://www.brucelipton.com/resource/interview/mind-growth-and-matter.

Imagine that someone at work criticises you about something, which causes you to play small; you find yourself not speaking up in meetings, for fear of being criticised again. You may be diverting to old stories and fear-based beliefs and reacting in autopilot. When this happens, question it. It is how we transform through our blocks that matters; not how we fall, but how we rise. Have you ever been angry at a loved one and reacted to something they have said? You can hear yourself angrily regurgitating negative dialogue, and a part of your brain thinks to yourself, 'Who am I right now?' It is almost like the behaviour comes out uncontrollably.

You know those times when you feel disconnected within yourself, like no one is home? The days when you've driven home, and you can't even remember what streets you turned down to get there. In this state we are not present, it is harder to be flexible, and much more difficult to see our life from a higher perspective. We are typically dwelling on the past or overanalysing the future. It is also our least creative state.

Negative behaviours like fear, bullying, anger and even rage are often expressed when we are on autopilot. These are critical points in our lives when what we choose is what matters. And we **can** choose our reactions. Later on, in The Pineapple Effect chapter, we will go into greater detail about how you can achieve this.

Top Tip!

Do you dry yourself after showering in the same way every day? Do you react to stress in the same way? Do you go to work on the same route every day?

Mix it up! Make it familiar to change your mind and behaviour about the smaller things. Make the unfamiliar, familiar. When you do this, it translates to the bigger changes you want to make for yourself in your life.

Living in the autopilot state

When we are stressed, we tend to focus on what we don't want: the negative and worst-case scenarios. In our modern way of life, we can get stuck living in a state of urgency, and long-term high levels of stress start to feel normal. Over time, high levels of stress impact on our health, our immune system, our thoughts and how we behave.

When we are stressed and typically not being the best version of ourselves, we can be reactive to people and our external environment. We know we are behaving badly, but we can't seem to control ourselves. That is because the belief we must protect ourselves becomes more dominant than the rational brain; we seem to lose the ability or will to change our mind about what we are believing in that moment.

When we vibrate at this lower frequency, we can stay in situations that aren't right for us. We can feel like we need alcohol or cigarettes to cope and, thanks to cognitive dissonance[11], we keep replaying the same pain and drama by attracting in more negativity. This is what makes us so tired, what causes so much stress, and why understanding our inner conflict can be the key that unlocks our barriers to wellness.

The good news is that there are practical things you can do each day to catch yourself when you are in autopilot. For instance, having daily morning and evening rituals is a great way to help us set our focus, to be more conscious and aware. When we go through a setback, trauma or a big change in life, we want to be particularly diligent to shift ourselves back into a present and calmer mindset. This will help us to operate from out most creative state, allowing us to move through change with more flexibility.

---

11 - Cognitive dissonance is the state of having inconsistent thoughts, belief or attitudes, especially relating to behavioural decisions and attitude change.

> ## Can You Notice the Difference?
>
> I have a great trick to help you identify and understand the difference between the autopilot and honeymoon states. Autopilot is the state we can go into when stressed and 'on' all day. By contrast, when we switch 'off' it is like the feeling you have on holidays – you feel like your nervous system has switched off inside you. Like a deep long exhale, aaaahhh!
>
> By letting go of our deepest fears and stresses, we finally feel safe enough to relax. We can also call this a rest, digest and nurture mode, as the brain is firing growth and repair signals. This is a pathway we want to prioritise, to heal; as opposed to feeling 'on' and wired in our heads, anxious and exhausted. Can you notice the difference?

When we are calmer and more present in the moment, we are happier, kinder and more adaptable to change. From this mindset, we can see our situation with fresh eyes, we can elevate our energy to be greater than our fears, seeing obstacles as opportunities with a new perspective.

The honeymoon state (the conscious)

The conscious brain is still powerful[12], despite it being in charge of approximately 5% of our processes and reactions. When we are in the moment and more mindful, we are in our most creative and innovative state.

Bruce Lipton explains how it works in his book, *The Honeymoon Effect*. Do you remember falling in love and being in that honeymoon stage? You are consciously thinking about what you are wearing, your etiquette, where your loved one is in the room. You are trying to show them the best version of you, and suddenly you are conscious of everything. They are too, and the energy of

---

12 - https://www.brucelipton.com/books/honeymoon-effect

two people mindfully creating consciously, being their best selves, feels amazing! But then life eventually gets in the way, we get stressed about the future and our jobs, and we are no longer present in the moment. We gradually become more and more familiar to each other. Over time, if we are not living consciously, more and more actions will be driven subconsciously. We can begin to think about the past or what we have to get done the next day, disconnecting and no longer experiencing that presence and connection together.

When we are in the moment and are mindful, we are not diverting to the subconscious program, which means we can literally create a new one. We are more adaptable to change, and this is when we can see more possibility. To transform our mindset and overcome any setback, we need to practise being more mindful, being in the moment, aware and awake. I call this 'living deliberately'. I like capturing this state in a morning and evening ritual that we will cover in a later chapter, and I also have a clever trick that helps me to bring myself back into the present moment, anytime I need to during the day. Because I am human, and I do forget.

A honeymoon or a more present state can be compared to the feeling you get when you are on holiday. You finally switch 'off', you give yourself permission to relax and wind down. This is how I felt when I came home from hospital. I was so grateful to be walking again and eating with two hands. Being able to drive myself independently to where I wanted to go. It made me so happy. I saw a whole new world through a fresh set of eyes. In this relaxed, joyful and grateful state, my body perhaps prioritised growth and repair, and this potentially was the catalyst for more healing.

That is why I am so passionate about being in a state that allows me to change my mind about what is possible, more open to managing change. We are typically in a conscious state for only 5% of each day, and I challenge you to make it much more.

When I learned how to align my (conscious) desires with what I was believing could be possible (subconscious belief), that is when the magic started for me. When I practised being more present, joyful and calm, I began to feel the joy of hope in all of my cells. When we do that, something shifts within us. This is the best environment we can give ourselves to overcome anything.

Living in the honeymoon state

When we are present and in the moment, we are calmer and in our most creative state. Catch yourself when you are focused on the past or addicted to thoughts that cause you to overanalyse the future. I wear a wristband that I designed that not only reminds me that 'I am enough', it also reminds me to catch myself when I am not being present, so I can bring myself back into the moment. I also catch myself in my reactions. If I feel my energy declining, I ask myself, 'What is this story I am replaying in my mind about? What am I believing about it? Is this story accurate, or is it an old one I am replaying from the past? Can I change my mind about it?'

It is in our best interests to be good at change. Because our bodies are designed to survive, being on alert and prioritising an alarmed state can dominate. When we become stressed, we tend to focus on what we don't want – the negative and worst-case scenarios – because this is the safest way. When our bodies are perceiving threat because of stress at work, at home or within relationships, we can react in a fight, flight or freeze response. Over a long period of time, this alarmed state can lead to inflammation and diseased states in the mind and body.

When we are calm, we are in our most creative and integrated state. When the brain no longer perceives that it needs to keep us safe, we can also give the mind and body the best environment to promote growth and repair pathways, rather than survival. When we are calm, we tend to focus on what we want, we can rise above the turbulence and see our life through new eyes, with a fresh perspective. We are more inclined to be kinder to others and ourselves, we find more motivation and will to overcome adversity, living happier and healthier lives.

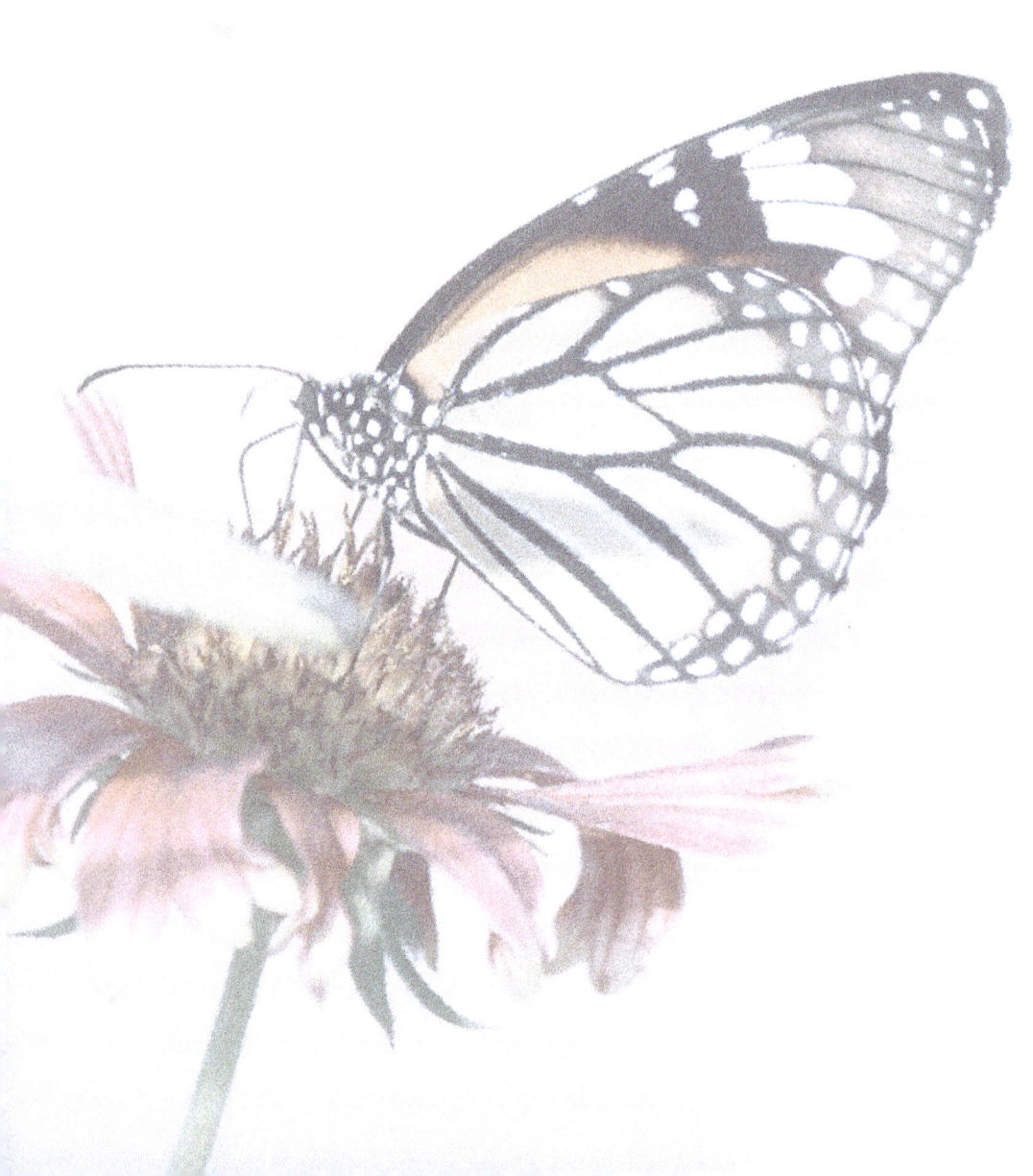

Chapter 4
What Causes Stress?

To understand resilience, we need to explore what causes stress. Stress is our response to a perceived threat (real or imaginary) to our security, mind or body. The stimulus may be external or internal. It may be physical, mental or emotional.

Our thoughts, emotions and vocabulary are all connected to our biochemistry. We typically operate from one of two pathways in the body: growth and repair or stress and survival. When we are stressed, the brain has perceived a threat and sent a signal out to our body to go into a state of survival, to protect us from danger.

A survival signal will fire hormones and neurotransmitters, such as adrenaline and cortisol, so that we can run faster from danger. When we feel safe again, we come back into balance, from being very 'on' to switching 'off', regulating our autonomic nervous system.

After an initial reaction of shock and alarm, we move into a stage of resistance. If we are stressed over a long period of time, it can lead into a state of burnout and exhaustion. Our digestion, brain integration, problem-solving skills and ability to heal all become compromised. Our brain is prioritising survival, instead of growth and repair. Illnesses like stomach ulcers, heart disease and nervous system issues are all stress-related diseases that we want to avoid. Long-term stress can be related to the suppression of the immune system. The body's organs show pathological changes, due to long exposure to stress hormones.[13]

---
13 - You can read more about the causes of stress in *Letting Go* by David R. Hawkins.

A time of stress for me

Back to my teenage years ... Nicole, my twin sister, immersed herself in Anthony Robbins' motivation work, listening to all his tapes (yes, back then they were tapes). She learned to rebuild her mind and saturated her cells with a liver cleansing diet that was popular in the 1990s. She began to rebuild herself.

I had finished Year 9 at Wesley College and didn't want Nicole to have to deal with a much bigger co-educational school on her first year back after taking nearly 4 years off. I found another school for us that was more suitable. By this time, the four of us (Mum, Muma, Nicole and I) had moved out of our family home, following my parents' separation. We set up a new home that was close to our new school, Strathcona, in the Melbourne suburb of Canterbury. It was a smaller school with an excellent academic education. We knew a few of the girls there which made Nicole's transition easier and as a result, she excelled. It was so great to have her back!

Deciding whether to pursue a career in music and dance (my passion), or whether to take an academic path, was a question I battled with throughout high school. I also loved the idea of studying law, as I did enjoy legal studies, and the concept of forensics fascinated me, but I didn't know myself or what I wanted. I started to subjectively develop ideas that I might be a disappointment, that I was not going to succeed in doing what I really wanted to do. I was loving music and the arts; my passion for music, singing and dancing got me through so many hard times as a teenager. For as long as I can remember, I had beliefs that I would not be successful, that it may be a battle for me to achieve what I wanted. I think that after so many years of living with chronic stress, not yet knowing how to optimise my mindset to be more confident and overcome these negative beliefs, contributed to a loss of confidence and self-esteem, which can also contribute to an inability to drive oneself forwards. I think I also lived with a lot of guilt because I was healthy, while Nicole had watched me live my life, at school and with new friends, without her.

In hindsight, I can now see that I should have pushed myself forward. I needed to find myself, despite the chaos going on around me. It was my path to learn who I was on my own and to develop enough love and confidence within myself, to understand who I was and what I wanted to do with my life, no matter what anyone else thought. But I had not grown to understand that yet. That requires a relaxation within, a rising and transformation that elevates us away from the anchors of our 'old story', so that we can create a new one.

When we are more still and anchored, we can begin to hear our inner guidance gently whispering 'this way'. When we are stressed, we overcompensate; for me, it was being in my head a lot and being very 'busy'. So I found myself holding back, thinking that pushing harder was the right thing to do. We make choices every single day, and every choice leads us onto another choice. Before we know it, all our choices combine and become the path of our lives.

In my teens and probably most of my 20s, I didn't believe I could do anything well enough. I was a perfectionist and very hard on myself. I got lost in the confusion, my high expectations and my inner critic, and I had an internal dialogue of 'you'll never make it'. I began to believe what I was hearing around me; I bought into other people's doubts, a fear mentality. I took this on and perhaps perceived the fears of the people around me, that they were not believing in me. But this reflected their stuff. I forgot how to be playful and loving towards myself. I had learned to disconnect so well. I didn't know how to control my mind to rise above my fear.

But I was always very driven and I never gave up. Despite my inner critic, I was determined and hungry to achieve. I was on a mission to 'make it' in my life, and I spent much of my adolescence wanting to show everyone that I could. The problem was, while I wanted so much, I did not yet believe that I could make it happen within myself. And so, an inner conflict was brewing within me.

We finished high school and Nicole absolutely killed it. Despite missing nearly four years of school, she had excellent grades for the remaining Years 10 to 12. I was mostly happy with my results, but I think I disengaged after Year 9 and didn't give it my all. My brain integration suffered, and I felt overwhelmed. I was falling behind in maths and accounting, subjects that contribute greatly to your final score. I didn't do as well as I had hoped, but not getting a university place into law or marketing eventually led me on a new path, to follow my dreams in music.

Initially I did enter my first year of university and studied Arts, majoring in Criminology to get a taste of law. It was fun. Nicole attended about 60% of the classes, but still needed more time at home to recover from her symptoms and anxiety.

We figured life was too short, and within a year took the plunge to follow our dream of singing and dancing full time. Nicole found a school called Dance Factory in Richmond, and we studied Music Theatre and Dance, learning jazz, ballet, tap and contemporary dance. We started to sing and wrote our own music, co-working with songwriters and producers we found via friends along the way.

We worked with producers and artists like David Higgins, Mark Rachelle, Sarah Godden, Israel, Vince Deltito from the famous old school talent show before *The Voice* was born, called *Young Talent Time*. We worked with their producers Anthony and David Tymo and had a ball; we just adored that crew. Nicky Whelan, now an actor living in LA, was one of the girls we met at Dance Factory; she became a close friend in our early 20s and was a big part of our journey in the music and dance scene. She introduced us to Mark Rachelle, a talented producer who we spent many years writing music with, down at the coast in Rye, Melbourne. I have such amazing memories from that era. We were doing what we loved, we felt alive, and it was amazing.

In my teens and 20s, while I didn't seem to have a problem going for what I wanted in my life, there was that inner conflict within me, holding me back.

As I touched on in the last chapter, there are events and changes that will come in our lives that push us out of our comfort zone and inevitably cause stress. When our nervous system perceives threat, it is not always from what you would think, such as living with an illness, accident, financial stress, death or divorce. We can perceive threat and react in a stress response from an experience of abandonment, interpersonal relationship issues, a lack of connection within ourselves or our tribe at home, within our friendships or our relationships at work. From how we feel about ourselves and our sense of belonging.

We can experience stress and perceive threat in our own individual and unique way, according to our life experiences, our environment, our circumstances, thoughts and beliefs. For me, my ability to be successful, to achieve and to experience an external sense of approval felt like a matter of life or death. I know now that what I needed to do, with a calm and more present mindset, was to challenge this story I had told myself. Was it true? Could I change my mind about what I believed? Could I align my goals with more positives beliefs about myself and what could be possible?

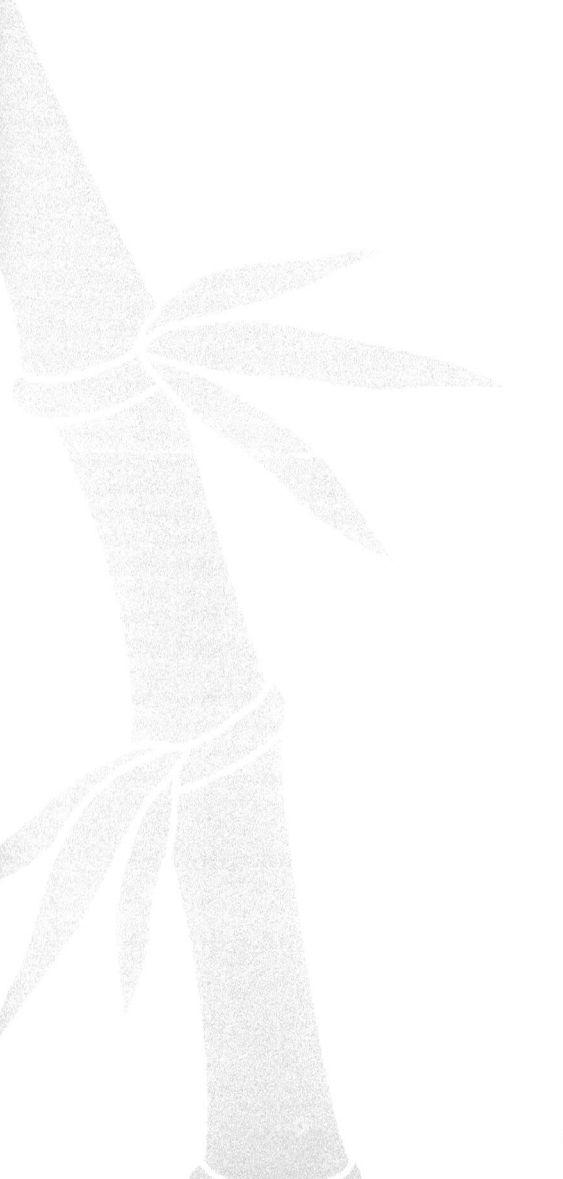

Barriers to wellness

We can get addicted to being busy and then it becomes familiar to function from this alarmed state – our least creative state. Becoming more aware of my blocks to wellness, and from observing patterns in clients at my private practice, it has been amazing to observe common denominators underlying what can make us tired, stressed, in pain (physical and emotional), or unable to promote healing and repair in our minds and bodies.

We have already explored the connection between our beliefs, how we perceive our reality, and how this alters our biochemistry. When we are stressed, we tend to focus on worst-case scenarios to protect ourselves. This affects how we perceive our environment, our reactions and our health.

We are designed to survive, and this is important, especially when we legitimately want to get out of danger, as when early man or woman needed to run from a predator. In our modern world with our modern problems, such as issues with finances, divorce and relationship issues, we can still respond by perceiving a real life-or-death situation, depending on how we perceive that stress.

We can also promote a stress response from drinking too much coffee, which signals our brain to fire adrenaline. In balance this can be fine, but if we are very stressed or anxious, it can just add more fire to the storm. We can also feel stressed watching the news and for some of us, this is how we start our day. How do you start your mornings?

Other stress can come from acute trauma or accidents. Or long-term stress, that tends to brew over a period. It feels like an inner resistance within yourself; you can't seem to put your finger on the cause, but you often know it's there, something just doesn't feel right.

Starting new projects, relationships, schooling or a career can create a stress response. Break-ups, death and the ending of relationships commonly induce stress that can trigger a fight, flight or freeze response.

Stress impacts our lives on a personal level in the following ways:

- Our mental health can be affected.
- We can overthink, suffering poor self-esteem and lack of confidence.
- A lack of connection with others and within ourselves can affect our relationships.
- Our ability to repair is compromised.
- We are not able to be as creative or innovative.
- It affects how successful and fulfilled we are.

Stress can also have an impact on our professional lives, depending on:

- how happy and healthy our culture is at work;
- how effective our productivity is at work;
- the bottom line, profit and business growth; and
- our ability to be innovative to effectively problem-solve.

I really love David R. Hawkins' explanation of the body's 3 nervous systems in his book, *Letting Go*:[14]

1. The voluntary network of nerves under conscious control and distributed primarily to voluntary muscles.

2. The involuntary or autonomic nervous system (sympathetic and parasympathetic), which is unconscious and controls the body's organs and physiological functions, such as heartbeat, blood flow/distribution, digestion and body chemistries.

3. The acupuncture system, which transmits bioenergy to all the body's structures and internal organs. This third system is least known in Western medicine but is long understood in Eastern medicine and society. In the acupuncture system, there is a flow of vital energies throughout the physical body via the body's invisible energy blueprint. This energy system is described as having 12 main channels over the surface of the physical body, down the 12 major acupuncture meridians. There are many tributaries leading from these channels into the body's various organ systems. Abnormal distribution of energy into these meridians results in dysfunction of the affected organs and muscles, and eventually the involvement of a disease process.

The vital bioenergy is the very flow of life itself and reacts very quickly to stress. The bioenergy reacts from instant to instant, due to fluctuating factors in our lives caused by the changing patterns of our perception, thoughts and feelings.

The brain decides which pathway to fire: one promotes growth and repair and the other fires a stress signal (prioritising survival), depending on how we perceive stress in our environment, past experiences and what we believe about ourselves and our circumstances.

---

14 - https://www.bookdepository.com/author/David-R-Hawkins

Our body will believe what we tell it. Our inner dialogue, and how we process and manage stress, plays a large role in whether the body chooses to prioritise survival pathways to keep us alive or chooses growth and repair pathways instead.

Barriers to overcoming stress

When I am consulting with clients, in the initial assessment I explore what is causing my client stress. We can find ourselves habitually living and reacting from a fight, flight or freeze response, perceiving that we are not safe. Some of us are addicted to this state so it can feel more familiar living wired and tired, than more grounded and present.

Eating a poor diet lacking in wholefoods and nutrients doesn't help either. In a stressed state, most people's digestive systems are not sufficiently nourished by minerals, vitamins and nutrients, which are critical not only for daily processes to occur, but also for our bodies to prioritise growth and repair. Throw in suppressed rage, anger, fear, low self-esteem, anxiety, overthinking and perceiving worst-case scenarios in our heads, which all activate a stress response within. When I am stressed, I am stuck in my head, I am unkind to myself and push myself harder. What helps me is having regular access to nature and the elements to naturally balance my nervous system. Morning and evening rituals help me to self-regulate.

In a society where our work can define whether we belong, or whether we are enough, we can literally feel as though our life depends on the success of our projects. Some of us are desperately seeking real joy and satisfaction in life because we have lost touch with how to receive it and feel it. We are overworked and we go, go, go, forgetting to stop to smell the roses. To relax, digest and receive what is already good in our lives. The inner numbness can stop us from receiving any satisfaction and joy, then one day we realise we have forgotten what is feels like to be truly happy.

Sleep is another important matter to address, because it is through sleep that we process each day and repair our minds and bodies. If you are experiencing burnout or are riddled with anxiety, depression or mental illness, I highly recommend prioritising a good night's sleep. Reach out to practitioners, if you are having trouble getting to sleep; if you are waking at 1am or 3am, for example, these are organ times according to Chinese medicine. Kinesiology or acupuncture can help to balance any stress in the meridians that are connected to your glands, organs and nervous system.

Stress and the intensity of our busy world can make it harder to put the brakes on; our brain is perceiving that it needs to live in a state of urgency to protect us. I have fallen into the trap of wearing the 'busy badge of honour' myself, because it made me feel like I was moving forward and away from a fear of not doing or being enough. Coming from a place of 'not enough' activates a busyness that is far from productive. It is usually an illusion that we are creating momentum, because often we are just stressed and regurgitating action. Being busy can also be a great way to suppress how we really feel about our circumstances or ourselves.

Perception is key. We can change our minds about what we are believing. We can trigger off an alarmed state just by thinking about the future or the past. A recent study conducted by neuroscientists at the Iran University of Medical Science[15] showed that this can also occur when kids play combat video games.

I am much more productive when I have a quiet mind, feeling grounded and connected. From this space, we can

---

15 - https://www.ncbi.nlm.nih.gov/pmc/articles/PMC6037427/

access more inner guidance, we can go with the flow, we can trust the process. Efficient productivity is knowing when to say 'no', what to walk away from, what to cull.

Therefore, my first step in assisting clients is to get to the bottom of what is stressing them out. I get them used to noticing a stressed state from a relaxed one, and we discover techniques that can help them put the brakes on in their minds, bodies and lives. I believe that the body can communicate to us with physical symptoms as a way of saying, 'Hey, pay attention! You are ignoring or suppressing unprocessed emotions or how you really feel.'

The negative impacts of being busy and in a stressed state long term include:

- ✘ decrease in the growth and regeneration of cells
- ✘ increase in inflammation and stress
- ✘ less brain integration and heart-brain-soul connection
- ✘ increased sense of urgency to rush and control, wanting more, never satisfied
- ✘ negative impact on learning, creativity and overall cognition

Some examples of modern and primal triggers for an alarmed and stressed state are:

- running from a predator
- war zone and lack of food
- meeting with an angry boss
- worrying about your family's finances
- caring about what people think
- worrying about letting people down
- being too fearful to walk away from a relationship that is not serving you

- feeling scared about your wellbeing and health
- being unemployed for months and worried you cannot pay your bills
- being hit with a lawsuit that threatens you financially
- going through combative divorce
- enduring major illness and feeling helpless
- feeling judged by your family or close circle of friends

What you can do about it

Because our bodies are designed to survive, we don't have to practise being good at 'survival mode'. What can be helpful is to practise feeling connected, more present and safe. Feeling more relaxed, we are better at letting go of stress, we can change our minds about the stories we tell ourselves, and we can boost our confidence and self-esteem.

Remember that coffee stimulates the adrenal glands and while it can be beneficial for relieving fatigue, too much of it can lead to anxiety and stress. Reducing coffee intake can be helpful if you are drinking a few cups a day. Consciously managing our stress levels and shifting into a calmer state can create a change in our biochemistry. I believe this is the best environment we can give ourselves to heal and adapt to change.

Our cells and biochemistry are connected to how we perceive our environment. We perceive our environment by referencing past experiences and what we believe to be true. If a negative belief causes stress, it will be a trigger for you. For example, let's say Person A believed they were confident and capable. One day, someone at work challenged their marketing presentation. Feeling confident, they would be more inclined to be open to how they could improve their presentation, making it the best it can be. They do not doubt their ability, and are thankful for the feedback. It's a non-event. People like this are great to debate with, because their response is constructive and this allows you to both learn from each other, rather than it being an emotionally triggering event that consumes too much unnecessary energy. Amazing leadership and innovation can come from these kinds of interactions and emotional wellbeing.

Now let's look at the example of Person B, who experiences the same situation. Person B doubts their ability and has low levels of confidence so might react emotionally, feeling angry and defensive, because they interpreted the criticism as an insult. They may feel dejected and downcast, seeing this as evidence that they aren't good at their job, or for that matter, at anything. When in fact, all that has actually happened is the marketing presentation was critiqued with a different point of view. These people are harder to work with, stunting creativity, innovation and productivity, especially in the workplace. It is unfortunate, because it means they will struggle to grow, professionally and personally. They are also not fun to work with.

You may have experienced both examples. The questions are: Who do you want to be and who would you prefer to be working or living with?

Have you ever experienced a heated reaction within yourself, where a comment has got under your skin and made you feel uncomfortable, for reasons you weren't able to pinpoint logically? Your reactions can give you clues about what you believe about yourself. These reactions often lead to an alarmed state, and therefore affect how we show up in the world.

There are two mindsets we can choose from. One asks: Why is this happening to me? I am not safe, let's push this change away! The other asks: How is this a mirror image of what is going on within me? How is this helping to teach me what I need to understand, so I can grow and become more?

The beliefs we create about ourselves are malleable; even our deeper, ingrained beliefs can be altered with a little work and repetition. How we think and feel, and what we believe and perceive in our environment, are connected to messages that are communicated to approximately 37.2 trillion cells in our body which determine what chemistry we fire: happy and restorative or inflammatory and degenerative.

Can you remove toxins and disharmony in your environment, such as:

- ✘ chemicals
- ✘ toxins
- ✘ toxic relationships
- ✘ medications and drugs (that are not right for you)
- ✘ violence
- ✘ junk food

Who and what you surround yourself with plays a big role here, so be mindful of:

- what you read
- your routines
- what you watch
- what you say
- your thoughts and inner dialogue
- how you feel
- your environment
- the kind of conversations you engage in

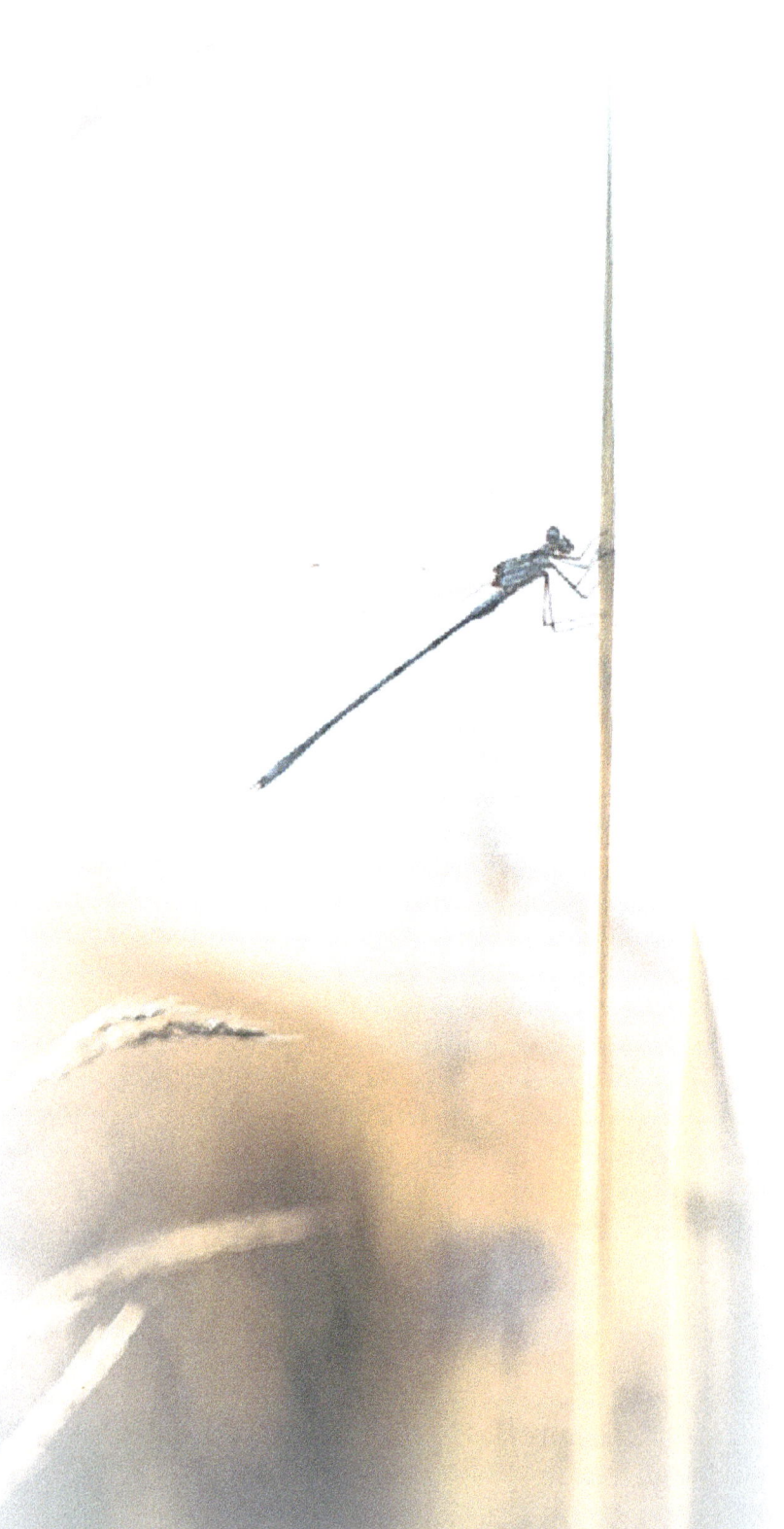

Chapter 5
What We Believe Is What Matters

In 2004, I was 24 years old and enjoying life in every way possible. We had stopped pursuing music as much and I was working in the fashion industry, a career that I loved. I was motivated, driven and happy. I had found a career I was good at, it stimulated me, I earned great money and I got to meet creative and interesting people. I worked at Sabatini Knitwear, initially as a receptionist, progressing within a few years to be Australian Coordinator. It felt like I was in the prime of my growing career and life. But my symptoms came back: pins and needles turned into weakness in my left arm, hand and leg.

I had another MRI, but this time I had my results analysed by a neurologist, a wonderful and kind doctor. On my way to meet him, I was in my 'coping Amanda' mode. Overcompensating, I replaced fear with an 'everything is fine' attitude. I was trying to be positive, but I was disconnecting. I thought that the MRI would show nothing. I was denying how frightened I felt about the appointment and its potential ramifications.

When I sat down with my neurologist, he looked at me, analysed my reports and said, 'Amanda, I am so sorry. Your results show that you have multiple scars on your brain, which means we can now diagnose you with multiple sclerosis. We can do a spinal lumbar puncture to confirm the results if you like. But in my opinion, it is conclusive, given you have multiple lesions in the brain.' He went on to explain that I had a few lesions on the right side of my brain, and one on my brain stem. A few years later, I would also find one on my spine.

Everything went into slow motion. I was shocked and didn't know how to react. I began to cry and asked him if I would be able to have a family one day. He told me that many people live on successfully, to be well and have families. I was lucky; I had a positive doctor who saw the glass half full. I am so grateful that he explained what could happen if my MS case ended up being 'benign', which meant there was a chance that my condition would not progress. But it also might, and there was no way of telling which way it would go. I nodded and to avoid being seen as vulnerable in a difficult moment, I ran into the next room and cried so hard I'll never forget it.

I was relieved that there was some hope, but I had no idea what MS really was or what I was facing. The unknown made me feel out of control, a feeling I knew too well and really didn't want to have back in my life. All my worst fears of not being successful or good enough suddenly came to the fore, and the news began to feel like my worst fears were coming true. I became more stressed and began to entertain what my life would be like if I ended up disabled, bedridden or worse.

MS is incurable, I learned. I thought there was nothing I could do to get better, except take the latest drugs, deal with the side effects, and just wait, hoping for the best. So, life felt like a ticking time bomb. I was fearful of my future and lived in an alarmed state, subtly but constantly. As a result, I didn't look after myself, and my actions and environment became an expression of how frightened I was. I began to believe deeply that I was not okay; I felt uncertain, alone and confused. I dove into work and kept myself busy to dull the emotional pain, frightened that my life and opportunities had a ceiling and time limit.

In such a state, we lose connection to our intuition and guidance. We are led by the monkey mind, solely by intellect that lacks intuitive guidance. No wonder things didn't feel like they were opening for me. Out of alignment, I started to believe that no one would ever love me, that I had nothing to offer of value anymore, that I may never have my own family, and may end up in a wheelchair, in some depressing nursing home.

Keeping busy became my overcompensation method, providing me with an escape. I am an extrovert at heart, so this suited me perfectly, as I found it quite natural to go into action mode to find answers. The keyword was 'trying', as my behaviour was also a mirror of my lack of trust in my future. I wanted to move forward, away from feeling so stuck, trapped, held back and out of control.

Feeling out of control is a common theme I have come across, when working with clients with MS and other neurological conditions of the brain. Because the brain is the control centre of the mind and body, emotional aspects of control (or perceiving to feel out of control in one's life) are often correlated and worked through in sessions.

If I am in action mode and problem-solving for solutions, being proactive is a trait that serves me well. However, when I'm out of balance it does not. I 'over try', I scramble, I have too many things on the go without doing justice to any of them. I lost focus as my mind was scattered across multiple processes; I overused my energy and created a self-sabotage pattern that made everything I was believing true. As a result, nothing really worked or gained the momentum I hoped for. I felt stuck, with no clear path forward. After living this way for several years, keeping myself overly busy, I was tired and my body started mirroring how emotionally paralysed I felt, leading to inflammation and stress in my mind and body.

Sabatini moved to Sydney, so I found a new role as a PA at J'Aton Couture, an amazing fashion house famous for made-to-measure couture gowns for brides and celebrities. The designers, Anthony and Jacob, were incredibly kind to me, understanding my health struggles. On my bad days, they would take over answering the door, so I didn't have to walk up and down the stairs too much – just gorgeous souls. I loved my job, and the boys were so talented and exciting. I fell in love with all the staff and felt lucky to learn from them. But I was not looking after myself, and I think it showed at times. I burned the candle at both ends, squeezing in every activity I could, in case my body failed me. And I paid the price.

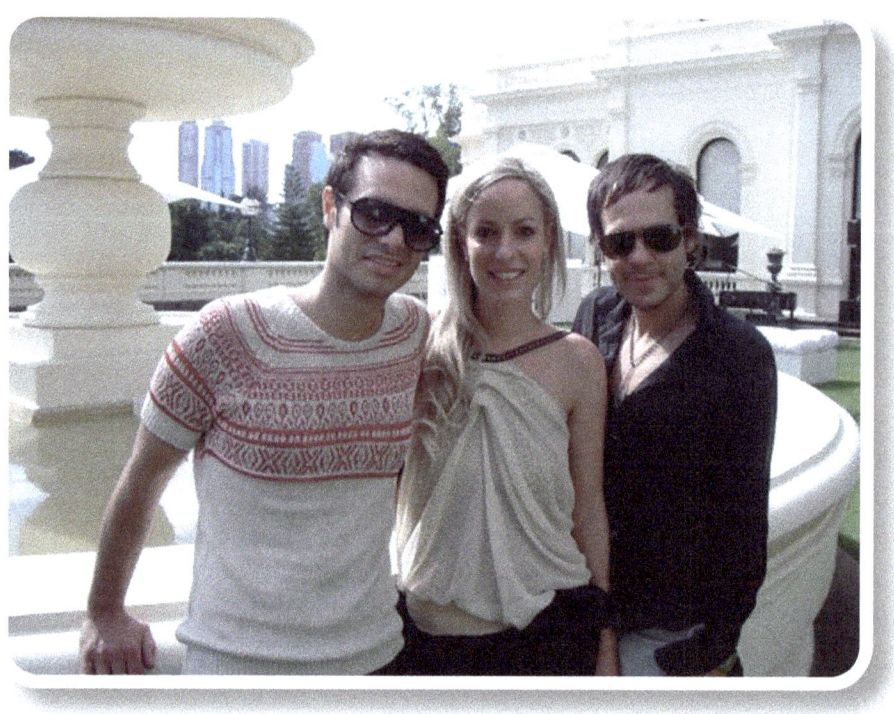

Jacob Luppino, Amanda & Anthony Pittorino from J'Aton

Now totally disconnected from myself and coping in the only way I knew how, I found it very hard to process and accept that I had MS. There were days when I just could not bear how I felt and had to escape my reality. So I went out later, worked harder, and disconnected more and more from my body, ignoring how I really felt about my future and having MS. It was too painful to feel that I may never achieve my dreams, that I may be unlovable or not enough, and therefore wouldn't experience life to the fullest. Deep in my heart, I always knew that I had a mission to achieve something in this life, but I was misperceiving that MS was a barrier to it, rather than the very catalyst that was to get me there.

It was easy to believe MS was a barrier. From a young age, I'd had negative beliefs about myself, so MS was simply the evidence my brain used to solidify those old ideas that became ingrained subconscious beliefs. That is what we do when we believe something: we look for evidence in our environment to prove that our beliefs are true, regardless of whether they are positive or negative. This can get us into trouble when we are stuck; we focus on what we don't want. We become stressed and entertain worst-case scenarios, then see our life through these lenses. When we make a conscious effort to focus on what we do want, and the positive, that changes everything. We notice more of what we are focused on, and we begin to feel happier and calmer. From this state, we can shift and change our minds.

But I was in my late 20s and feeling stuck. As a result, my reality was mirroring my thoughts; I was experiencing more inflammation, stress and chronic illness. And the worst was yet to come. I had some minor symptoms over the next few years, including numbness, balance issues, and weakness on the left side of my body. They were often years apart, so I continued to live my busy life, mostly in denial of my diagnosis.

In 2009, at 29 years of age, my worst fears were realised. Over a slow, cruel 10 days, the entire left side of my body was paralysed, a consequence of a new lesion on the motor skill area of the right side of my brain. If you drew a line down the middle of my face down to my pelvis, the whole left side of my body stopped working completely. I lost the ability to walk and life as I knew it. My body was mirroring how emotionally paralysed I felt within myself.

I couldn't work and lost my financial independence. I was forced to completely stop. Simple little things, like the ability to wash and feed myself, became the most difficult tasks of my day. I had been living my life totally focused on experiencing everything that I could, then suddenly found myself in turmoil and darkness. I felt totally helpless and out of control on a new level.

My sister had to literally drag me on her back, up and down stairs, along the carpet and into the car to urgently see my neurologist. He took one look at me, and I knew by the look on his face that he was thinking, 'Oh no!'.

They checked me into hospital in January 2009 and I knew I wasn't going to be leaving any time soon. They started me on the standard MS therapy, which is a high dose of steroids for three days. I didn't respond. They continued the high dose of steroids for another two days, five days in total, but I still could not move. It was the hardest and darkest time of my life.

I was transferred to rehabilitation within the hospital, and this is where the real work began. I hit rock bottom. I had to ask myself, 'Am I ever going to walk again?' I was stretched to my limits, emotionally and physically, beyond normal comprehension.

I had a meeting with the head of the rehabilitation department, who explained that they could not guarantee I would ever recover. I was faced with being permanently disabled at 29 years of age. And I began to believe that I wasn't going to be okay.

Our beliefs have a big impact

Have you ever noticed that just wanting something is not enough to make it happen? Have you also noticed that hard work can sometimes make things happen; but other times you can be working your butt off, but still feel like you are getting nowhere? That is because what we believe matters.

Our beliefs directly impact on everything in our lives. What we believe is connected to what we attract, the life we create, our perceptions, how we show up every day, as well as the health of our mind and body. What we believe will dictate:

- how we show up and the decisions we make;
- how we manifest things into our life, and our ability to create for ourselves; and
- the biochemistry we fire and the health of our body.

The brain's Reticular Activating System (RAS) looks for evidence in our environment that aligns with what we're focused on. Its job is to bring more resources to us, so we can create and make things happen for ourselves. I'll discuss the RAS in detail in a later chapter.

What we focus on depends on how stressed we are. When we are stressed, we tend to focus on what we don't want: in a fear state, we can entertain worst-case scenarios to protect ourselves. When we are calmer and able to be more present in the moment, we are adaptable to change, so we tend to be more open-minded and flexible, focusing on the positive.

For instance, when we are stressed, we are focused on what we don't want and worst-case scenarios, fear builds up inside us and we can feel exhausted. Fear can keep us playing small in our lives, in a sabotage loop. When we feel like this, we can think from a rigid mindset that leads to more unhappiness and poor health.

On my journey, I had to learn how to train my brain to focus on what I wanted, on feeling positive and motivated, so I could elevate my energy to overcome mental and physical degeneration. On days when I was feeling more connected, powerful, positive and strong, I could access creative solutions around me, and I noticed changes in my body.

I learned that when we have practised believing in ourselves and the positive, we are well-rehearsed to manage change and adversity when they come. We can see our setbacks as opportunities. We are more inclined to get out of our comfort zone, to become our fullest potential.

When we believe in ourselves and what can be possible for us, our goals can align with our inner beliefs. Because of this alignment, it is easier to make things happen. We can focus on what we want and best-case scenarios. We are more imaginative, creative and innovative. The most incredible thing I discovered about this alignment is that it can also create more harmony in the body, promoting repair.

When I was paralysed, I was in a situation where I had no choice but to change my mind about what I was believing, to get different results. Adversity can be an opportunity for us to create change in our lives and discover what we are made of.

Without the use of my body for a month, I very quickly learned about the power of my mind. I did a lot of work on my belief systems and really had to face up to a lot of truths.

This wasn't easy and was sometimes quite confronting. However, the stakes were high and I knew that I had to make important changes, to get better results.

After about 6 weeks of paralysis, my toe finally moved. This ignited such hope and joy that something really shifted within me. I became clear about what I wanted, instead of what I didn't want. I reconnected back into my body, I got out of my head and dropped back into my heart. From there, everything began to change rapidly.

In the short term, I noticed that I began to repair faster. In the long term, my whole approach to living changed. I went from being in a wheelchair, to having a foot brace, to having my knee taped up, to walking on my own. And those first steps walking again were indescribable!

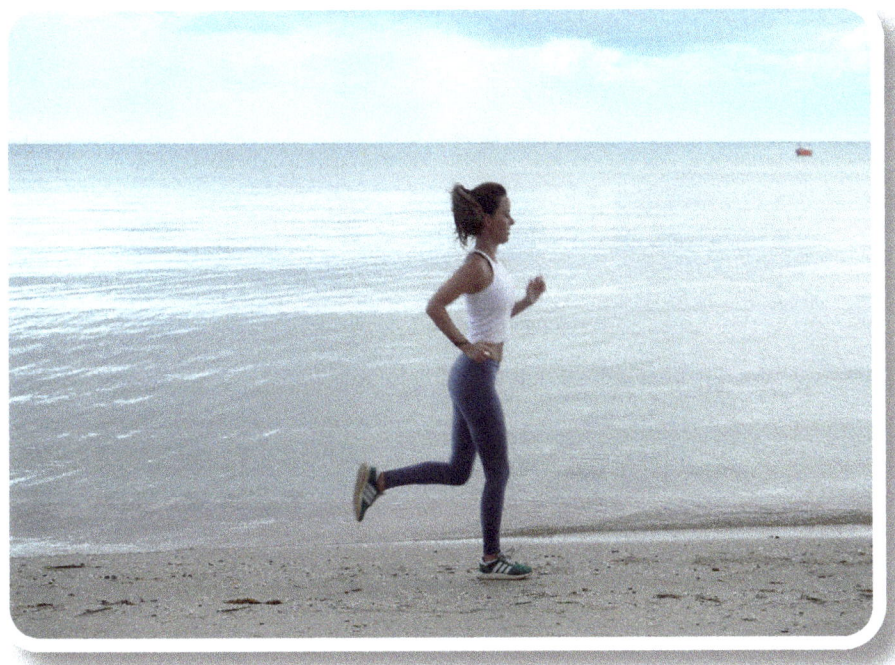

Amanda running on the beach

My experience taught me that my mindset is directly linked to the health of my body. When we use our energy to give the mind and body the best environment to be flexible and resilient, we are calmer, we are more present, we are less rigid to change, and we are more adaptable. When we are feeling good, we can let go of old pain, shifting out of stress into growth and repair instead.

We cannot control change, but we can control how we react, how we perceive our environment, and therefore how stressed we become.

How you can believe

What we believe is like a projection screen that creates our reality. It mirrors the people who show up in our life and they are a mirror of what we need to look at within ourselves. Before you judge, ask yourself: What is this situation showing me? What am I to learn here? What needs to be healed within me, that I may not be acknowledging or taking responsibility for?

The good news is that you can stop searching externally! Go within, all you seek is within; access that and master it. Feel your body again, drop out of the head and into your heart – then keep it open. Let go of the need to protect yourself; you now have the tools to anchor yourself, you are more flexible, you can master change. Find the courage to feel safe enough to experience all your emotions; they all serve you. Learn to control your mind and your stress levels.

There is no end point, there is only an ongoing journey of learning. Sometimes we will have amazingly joyful times, and sometimes more difficult times. Sometimes life will bring soul-searching chapters that take us to the next level. I think that every time we grow, we elevate to the next level in our life. As we progress, we will see with a higher understanding, the light will become brighter with expanded awareness, and the understanding that comes with that will overwhelm you with joy.

Without polarity, the light and dark moments, there would be no understanding. Knowing despair allows us to receive and understand joy. Expect setbacks, expect change, don't fight it, lean in. Swim downstream into the current, surrender and let it take you. Expect best-case scenarios, focus on what you want, notice more positivity around you. You can choose to believe you have found your inner anchor to protect you – you've got this. On the other end of this ride, a new world and dimension awaits; a new you and a life more amazing than you can even comprehend.

We are always on a path to becoming. I recommend that you pull back, do less, stop trying so hard, as this comes from a place of lack. When you begin to believe in yourself and what can be possible for you, you will just know your next move; you will trust that you have the resources that you need for your chosen path.

To create a new mind, body and life, we must become a whole new version of ourselves. Our thinking, our vocabulary and our actions can all adjust, when we change our minds about what we have been believing in the past. We must get out of the old story, out of our own way, and see the past with fresh eyes, elevated and with fresh insight.

In my earlier life, I believed that I needed more help, support and connection, believing it was missing from my life. I didn't know how to experience this within myself, and it became so limiting. But I know now that illness, break-ups and other setbacks were obstacles perfectly placed to enable me to discover these virtues within myself. So that I could change my mind about what I was believing, and therefore my perception. I remember the day I woke up, looked in the mirror, and realised that I had found my power. I finally felt so deeply connected, loved and supported, after believing this was lost for much of my life. Our beliefs can transform, and they must do so; I believe this is the point of life.

We have all had events that have hurt us. Let go of your old story. Painful memories can serve us if we learn from past mistakes. But when we get stuck in the pain and overthink and identify with the story too much, it can become a burden and a problem. This is called 'hell on earth'; we stay stuck in a prison, reliving the old pain. Then every future thought, perception and action just serve to relive the past, which means we cannot create a new future, mind, body and life for ourselves. We limit ourselves when we hold onto shame, guilt, anger, fear, jealousy and worry.

Can you bend and get out of your old story? Let it go. Change your mind and see it from an elevated perspective, giving the past a new meaning. You might find yourself begin to perceive it differently, freeing you from your jail. You will be in the same environment, but everything will look different, more beautiful, more colourful. Welcome to heaven on earth when you elevate and see the light again!

Can you listen more? If you can just surrender a little bit more, you will understand that you are fully guided the whole way. Learn to listen to your body, empty and wash the mind regularly. This is your compass, to help you reconnect to who you really are.

We can catch ourselves when we are disconnected, when we have checked out, living in autopilot. When we find ourselves stuck in the past or overanalysing the past or the future. Remember that I mentioned using a wristband to catch yourself in negative moments? This is a trick I know you will learn to love as much as I do!

Our reactions are a mirror of what we are believing. Check in with your reactions, they can be a clue to help you get in touch with your inner beliefs, exposing any inner conflicts that may be out of your awareness. Our beliefs and perceptions are malleable; we can change our minds about what we are believing and therefore about what can be possible for us.

Our health is a mirror of what we are thinking, feeling and believing. If you are dealing with physical symptoms, you can use a mind-body approach, with the help of kinesiology, to uncover underlying beliefs and blocks that may be linked to your symptoms.

You can rewrite your story. Bring awareness to your reactions, to uncover the underlying beliefs you have about yourself and what is possible for you. With this awareness, you can begin to change your mind about what you are believing.

We can review our perceptions. An old idea may not align with the wisdom you have now. If you are feeling reactive, challenge your beliefs. Changing your perspective can create a shift in how you see your world.

These mindset hacks can help to empower you to reset your focus, to live more in the present moment, our most creative state. With flexibility and a resilient mindset, you will feel ready, anchored and confident.

No matter what you are going through, I want you to believe that you can overcome it. Feeling more resilient, you can begin to expect best-case scenarios; then you will notice more energy, willpower and vitality in your mind and body. With an elevated mindset, you can begin to see obstacles as opportunities to grow, so you can become a new version of yourself that is more open to healing, joy, love and your fullest potential.

Chapter 6
The Power of the Mind

My first symptoms …

At age 19, when we weren't studying and dancing at Dance Factory, Nicole and I worked at Chasers Nightclub to earn money. One night, I felt numb on the left side of my face. I remember arriving for my shift at the VIP lounge upstairs, I was running late, applying my mascara using the mirror behind the spirit bottles on a lower shelf. I noticed that I couldn't feel the mascara as I applied it to my left eyelashes. While I was talking to my boss, Bec, drool was coming out of the left side of my mouth. I apologised and put my hand up to my lips to catch it, giggling with embarrassment. The numbness gradually extended to my left arm, fingertips and foot. I was shaken and booked in to see the doctor.

My family GP was concerned that my symptoms could be from a brain tumour or something neurological, so he sent me off to have an MRI. I was terrified about putting 80% of my body into a tunnel of doom for 45 minutes. I had to brace myself with a light sedation to get it done.

To this day I do not enjoy an MRI, but thankfully the tunnel is getting bigger as they produce new ones, which makes the experience much more manageable. It helped enormously when Scott, my partner at the time, came in to hold my feet, making funny faces to distract me. I loved him for it.

Back to when I was age 19, the MRI showed one lesion on the right side of my brain, but there was no solid prognosis or diagnosis. It turns out we can get white plaques and spots on our brain, that are sometimes inconclusive and nothing to be concerned about. True to my nature, I just got on with my life. I was a doer, so I did what I knew and went into action. I kept myself busy with work, using fear as my driver to try harder in life. I didn't process the difficult emotions, as I didn't know how to, so I suppressed a lot of my fears.

In my early 20s, my twin sister Nicole and I worked hard on our music, and we wanted to go all the way in our career. We had meetings with a few record labels. I managed to get us an interview with Sony, at the time when Rogue Traders was getting big (an electronic rock band, featuring Natalie Bassingthwaighte). The Veronicas (Brisbane-born identical twin sisters, Lisa and Jessica Origliasso) were also launching their career as artists in the industry. Music was such a large part of our lives in the early 2000s. It was such a fun time, and we were on the path to live the life we wanted. Still, it wasn't easy.

Looking back, I know now that our outcomes are affected by how much we believe in ourselves; as it turns out, we didn't believe in ourselves enough. We were still recovering from what we had been through, figuring out our unique superpowers and how to propel ourselves forward with confidence. We'd had the willpower to get through so much stuff in the past, but as young adults, it's as if we were too burdened by whatever anchored us into a sabotage pattern we'd never quite broken out of.

I didn't know it at the time, but my fear of failing and being criticised became my biggest setback and dominant program. Because of that, I made decisions that kept myself small. Everything became a mirror of what I believed about myself: that I wasn't successful enough or good enough. I didn't yet understand that I could question those beliefs, and it never dawned on me that they might not be true. I quickly learned to shut off and suppress my difficult emotions, and I became excellent at just 'getting on with it'. A master, in fact. I used my drive and focus, disconnecting more and more from my body, my emotions and my pain.

Looking back, I can see that some of the hurdles Nicole and I had to go through with illness and stressful life events had activated an alarmed state within me, that never really switched off afterwards. When we go through a difficult time that causes stress in our lives, this 'on' switch can stay on as a protective mechanism. As a result, I think I saw the world through lenses of fear, focusing most of my energy on protecting myself. This stressful state doesn't allow for a flexible mindset, where I may have been able to let go of the past, changing my mind that I was safe, I was loved, and that I was good enough. I created a reality around me that mirrored my fears, and it was all completely out of my awareness.

Learning to go within

Spending a few months unable to use the entire left side of my body taught me about the power of my mind. I had so much time on my hands and experienced moments of stillness that I previously had never dared to entertain, due to painful and unprocessed emotions. With no choice but to sit with myself and within four white walls, I had to go within. After a lifetime of searching for guidance, answers and personal power externally, I began to discover inner resources that were activated from my experience of being paralysed that I had to throw out all my old ideas, habits and beliefs.

I learned about the power and importance of our inner anchor. Once accessed, it is incredible what we can achieve. From there, I could regulate an inner power that I felt I had always had access to. But it was not quite activated until I had no choice but to go within; then I was forced to get reacquainted with just how powerful I could be.

Without the use of the left side of my body for nearly two months, I quickly learned about the power of my mind. As I began to shift what I was believing, and I could see better results, I had more motivation and courage, and I began to repair faster.

I believe that flexibility builds resilience. A flexible mindset can optimise our health and our lives. This is critical when we are going through change and transformation. The health of our mindset can determine the decisions we make, how we react while solving problems and inevitably, the health of our bodies. The mind-body connection is powerful. A flexible mindset impacts on everything that matters: our body's ability to repair; how happy and resilient we are; and how connected we feel within ourselves, and to others.

Athletes know that when we are mentally rehearsing a movement routine in our mind, the brain can't distinguish whether the movement is happening now in real time, or if the mental rehearsal is just a thought. Brain scans have shown that thought alone can create a similar pathway in the brain as occurs when the exercise is being performed. How incredible is that!

How we think and feel is a reflection

Our mindset is a mirror image of what we believe about ourselves. How we think and feel is a mirror image of what:

- we see in our own reality
- occurs electromagnetically in our Qi (energy) system
- occurs biochemically in our body
- occurs physically in our body

Imagine you woke up anxious. That feeling would present structurally, biochemically, emotionally and energetically, both simultaneously and in an integrated fashion.

Structurally: Our posture changes because the tension of our muscles alters with stress, and with the different emotions we experience. For example, when sad or stressed we might be slouched over, mirroring a closed heart, protecting ourselves. Our pelvis can rotate because of a change in tension in our hip muscles. We may experience lower back pain if we are holding onto something in our lives that no longer serves us; it can be a state of guilt, grief or longing.

Biochemically: We have all experienced the relationship between how we feel and our digestive system, the bladder and even our bowels. The amygdala gland of the brain is involved with our emotional responses, such as anger, fear, enjoyment, love and joy, and there is a direct correlation to how our organs perform. For example, constipation or diarrhoea can occur because of unprocessed emotions, because our emotions are connected to our organs.

In traditional Chinese medicine, the philosophy cleverly and accurately connects different emotional states to different organs. This is how kinesiologists work with the body; acupuncturists use the same 5 element system too.

How we feel, together with our posture, affects how our mitochondria converts food into energy, how our organs assimilate nutrients and minerals, the expression of our hormones, our neurotransmitters, and how our brain fires. When we are stressed, we often crave carbs or sugar, alcohol or substances. Other biochemical aspects that can also be considered are toxins, viruses, bacteria, infection and genetic expression.

Emotionally: We can feel joy, anxiety, anger, sadness, fear, guilt, shame, pensiveness, worry or craving, just to name a few emotions. If we have been stressed for a long period of time, we can also experience disconnection, attempting to escape these lower vibration emotions that feel overwhelming. You know how it feels, when you are stuck in a rut and it's hard to be inspired enough to get out of it or visualise how to execute a new direction. Willpower, joy and courage are important higher vibration emotions, that help to propel us out of these states. Even anger can be an important emotion to propel us forward out of sadness, for example. Balancing our emotional wellbeing can promote balance in our bodies physically, biochemically and spiritually.

Energetically: This is energy, our life force, our Qi. It can be felt when holding acupoints, similar to the sensation of a pulse of the blood. The health of the flow of our Qi affects our behaviour. For example, when our kidney Qi is depleted, it may affect our willpower to move forward. In traditional Chinese medicine, our kidney organ is related to the virtue of moving forward with wisdom and willpower. An emotion that blocks the kidney flow is fear, which affects how inspired we feel. Our gallbladder Qi is directly related to our ability to execute our plans and is connected and related to the liver organ. When we are suppressing anger, a dominant emotion in the liver and gallbladder it can cause procrastination. Because anger is an outwardly directed emotion, it can propel us forward. Anger can serve to disperse a procrastination pattern, if it is not violent or expressed with the intention to hurt others.

Kinesiologists work to create balance of Yin and Yang Qi running through the meridians. Our energetic bodies are more malleable that our physical, which is why creating flow in our Qi can create relief in body pain and can realign our posture. Our energy systems are connected to our bodies physically via our muscles, tissues, tendons, ligaments, fascia and nerves.

The link between pain and emotion

Physical symptoms are often an end result of not listening to our inner voice, that guides us to know what is right or wrong for us. Working with clients at my private practice, when I began analysing common symptoms, I discovered patterns. For example, if someone who suffers from a sore neck and shoulders is not getting any relief from physical adjustments, like physio, chiro or massage, that can indicate that the source of stress needs further investigation. What I love about kinesiology is that we can assess the body as a whole, then search for the source of stress on all levels: structurally, biochemically, emotionally and energetically.

Many of the neck muscles are related to the spleen and stomach meridians, and a trained Chinese medicine practitioner can investigate how a patient is feeling emotionally. Clients with neck pain can have links to suppressed emotions of pensiveness[16], worry and overthinking. Consequently, they are unable to close the loop of their minds as they go over and over the past or the future, in order to cope. This closes the heart and fear rises in the body up to the chest, sometimes creating heart palpitations, triggering more stress and a protective state.

What we believe is what matters. If we are living in our heads and overthinking, rather than in a calm and compassionate state of heart, it is like seeing through lenses of worry and fear, perceiving more threat around us. We

---

16 - Pensiveness is when one is brooding about life or a situation, constantly or obsessively overthinking about life, rather than living it.

are more reactive and less creative, and more symptoms surface from this accumulation of stress and energy, so the cycle goes on.

When this information is connected and brought to the client's attention, we can then look at how it may be playing out in their life currently, and when it started. This helps us dissect the pattern and find the cause, addressing the body as a whole rather than in isolation.

Addressing the body in an integrated way means we can look at all layers of the physical, emotional, biochemical and spiritual aspects of the client, when correcting physical pain. A physical correction could be a trigger point to relieve the pain in the muscles. Some other structural aspects of the body are organs, facia, tendons, ligaments, tissues and nerves. Identifying an emotion that is out of balance can help to shift tension and stress physically because, as we are learning, the body is so connected.

From there, we can target relevant organs, glands, systems of the body and the biochemical pathways that may be involved. We can identify specific nutrients that can support the body to promote repair. When we address the body electromagnetically, we can move the Qi to create flow in the mind and body, by touching (or needling with acupuncture) acupressure points on the body.

Pain in the lower back can be related to the emotions of not letting go, holding onto stuck grief, guilt or sadness. Dealing with the emotional link to the physical ailment can be like turning the tap off at the source. It is so amazing that our physical symptoms can be an end result of unprocessed thoughts and emotions. Could this be our bodies way of saying, 'Pay attention to how you are feeling or what you have been ignoring'!?

I regularly blog about the emotional links to physical stress and diseases in the *Bend Like Bamboo* blog.[17] You can

---

17 - Check out my website: https://www.amandacampbell.com.au/blog

also find videos on my YouTube and podcast also called *Bend Like Bamboo,* as well as many free resources on my website.

Chapter 7
The Mind-Body Connection

Our thoughts, emotions and vocabulary are all connected to our biochemistry. When we are stressed and the brain perceives a threat, it sends out a signal to our body to go into a state of survival, to protect us from danger. In days gone by, a life-or-death situation could have been running from a tiger to stay alive. In such a situation, we'd switch into 'survival mode' which is a stress response. Our bodies are designed to survive; our brain's priority is to keep us alive.

A survival signal will fire adrenaline and cortisol out to our body, so we can run faster to keep from danger. When we feel safe again, we switch out of 'survival mode' into a 'rest, repair and digest mode', to balance our autonomic nervous system.

The stresses of modern-day living such as finances, relationships, divorce, change, illness, or just watching the news while drinking coffee, can all trigger off adrenaline and a stress response. The trouble is, after being 'on' for most of the day, many of us forget to take the time to switch 'off' and balance out our nervous system.

Although we have different stresses than in times gone by, we can still fire a stress response when dealing with modern-day hurdles. Our mindset and mental health also matters. When we continuously operate in a survival state, our immune system can become compromised over time. We can experience a loss in motivation and vitality, and our health may deteriorate. This is not the best environment to optimise repair or resilience. Many of us just don't realise that our thoughts, emotions and ability to manage stress are all linked to how well or unwell we feel. Therefore, learning how to switch off regularly can really help us to restore our wellbeing.

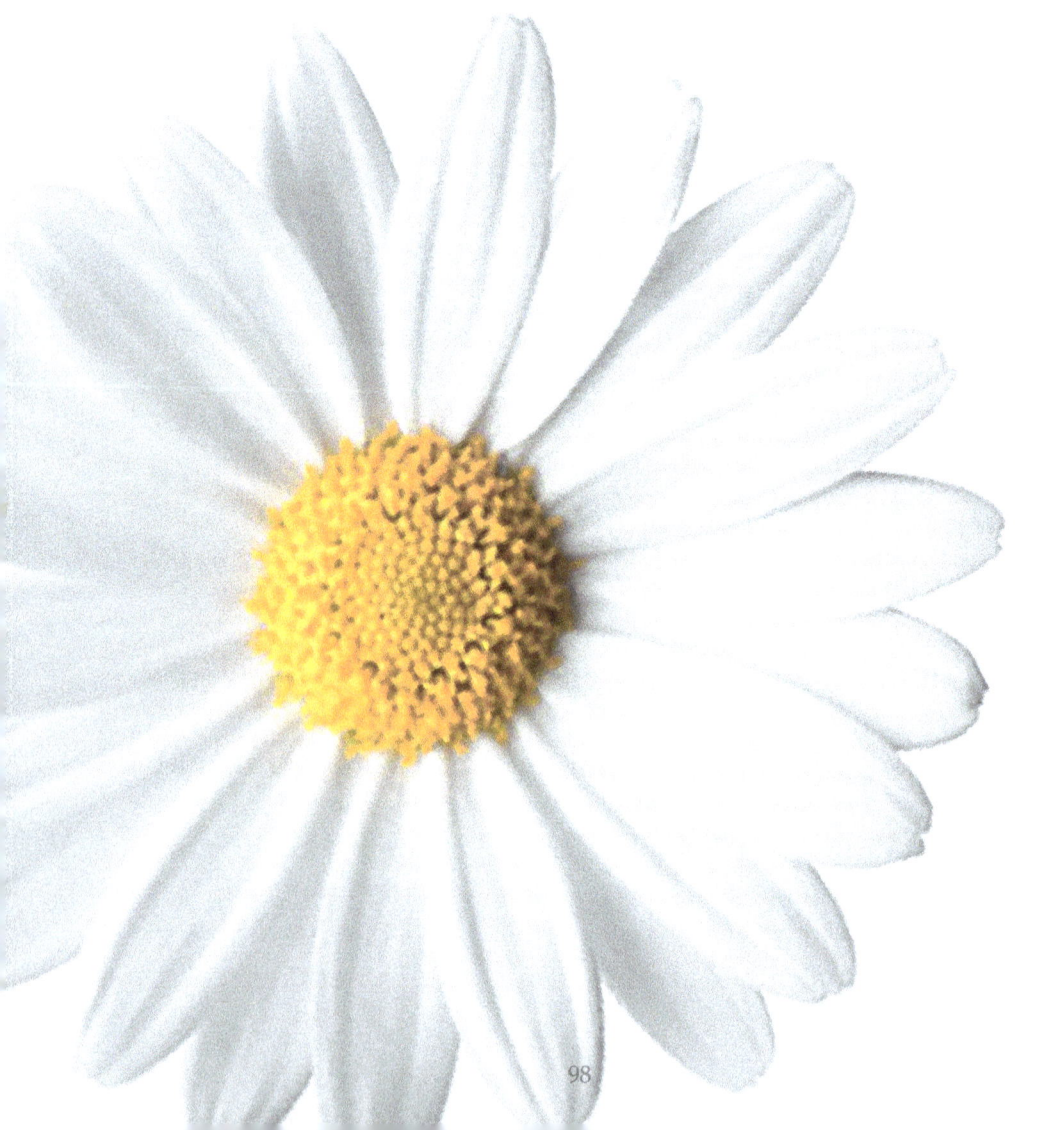

Identifying our beliefs by our reactions

How we think and feel and what we believe are so important and dictate how we perceive our environment, and therefore how stressed we can be. Often, negative and painful beliefs can be outside our awareness, as we become very good at pushing them away and suppressing them. Observing our reactions can help us understand what we believe about ourselves, how we are thinking and feeling about our circumstances.

When I was in my mid-20s, I was living in fear of my future. I started to believe that I had only a short time to enjoy my life, because of my MS diagnosis. As a result, both my outer and inner worlds mirrored these thoughts, which led to disconnection. I stopped looking after myself.

Five years later, at age 29, my worst fears were finally realised. I became paralysed because my disease had progressed, inflaming the motor skill area of my brain. My body began to mirror the inner mental turmoil I was feeling.

Now it doesn't always have to be as extreme as that. Look at your common reactions and trace back any connecting beliefs.

It is also helpful to notice physical states. For instance, do you get headaches or tummy aches? Headaches, neck aches, even shoulder aches are often linked to excessive worry, obsessive thoughts and fear.

Exercise: *Linking common reactions to beliefs*

Take a moment now to write down some of your common reactions. Then think about the beliefs that underpin or motivate those reactions. The good news is that when we practise catching our reactions, we can then question them. Each time we choose a new reaction, we can shift what we are believing.

This is how I learned to be more resilient on my journey. It was amazing, observing the changes as I chose new reactions. This led to more harmony in my body, and I felt happier as a result.

The mind and the body are so connected. Studies and clinical research show that the placebo effect is real and demonstrates the power the mind has over the body. For example, a group of women were told they would be given a hotline injection, to bring on their menstrual periods 2 weeks early. In fact, they were given a placebo injection of saline. Over 70% of the women developed early premenstrual tension, with all the physical and psychological symptoms.[18]

We have all experienced a physical or biochemical reaction in our bodies from thoughts and emotions. For example:

- **nervous** – we can feel tense in our stomach or bladder
- **excited or anxious** – we can feel butterflies in our gut, or a loss of appetite
- **sad** – physically, our posture slumps
- **worried** – we can experience sore neck and shoulders
- **not moving forward** – we can experience a sore lower back

---

18 - To read more about this research, see Letting Go by David R. Hawkins.

The lenses of life

How we think, feel and believe are also a mirror image of how we perceive our environment and our interactions. In other words, our thoughts are a mirror of how we interpret our reality.

When we want to optimise our health or if we want to boost resilience within our lives, it is important to give our body the best environment for it to choose repair and growth pathways. Inner dialogue is key: what we tell ourselves sends a signal to our cells. Our actions mimic what we believe, and we inevitably create more of the same in our environment around us. We subconsciously mirror our beliefs, making them true all day long. This is how the brain works.

We discussed our reactions and how they can give us a clue about what we are believing. Have you ever noticed that when you react negatively to something not going your way, it typically correlates with something else in your life that is not going as planned? For example, let's say you lost your keys and were late to work. Let's pretend you reacted by saying, 'Of course I lost my keys; one more bad thing to happen to me today!' This is a very reactive response, and is showing you what you are believing about yourself, and how you are perceiving stress in your life. Losing your keys simply triggered a negative belief in you that was already there and is an example of how an external trigger can lead to a reaction.

Such events are gifts, exposing what needs to be transformed within us, that we may have been suppressing for quite some time. Painful beliefs and emotions can be difficult to look at, but when left unacknowledged for too long, they can accumulate as excess energy, creating pain or inflammation in our bodies. Physical symptoms can also be a sign for us to dive deeper into what we are ignoring emotionally.

Let's flip the example and pretend you were in a positive place in your life, feeling confident, believing that things do work out for you. With this mindset, you may have reacted more like this: 'Oh, bugger! I lost my keys,' and the reaction would have ended there, not getting under your skin. Learning how to remain calm and anchored within ourselves allows us to effectively problem-solve, so we can notice more creative solutions around us.

It is amazing how much energy we use, getting triggered by our beliefs and reactions. However, we can pick up clues from our reactions; they can show us what we are believing. With that awareness comes choice and the ability to challenge our thinking, habits and dialogue. With this awareness we can feel empowered to overcome our challenges creating positive change in our lives.

When we are more present in the moment, mindful and conscious, we can create new ideas, more positive beliefs and responses. When we are calmer, we are in our most adaptable state forming the lenses that we see our life through.

The reticular activating system

The reticular activating system (RAS) is a formation of nerves deep within the brainstem.[19] It acts as a filter, separating out unnecessary information so important messages get through.

Whatever our focus is, we will see more evidence of that in our environment. If you believe that you are not enough, it is like putting on glasses and seeing through lenses that only allow you to see things that represent 'not enough'; everything around you will appear this way, altering how you think and feel. The good news is that we can leverage the way the brain works to shift our focus from the negative to the positive, leading to an optimistic mindset and better outcomes in our lives.

Start with your inner dialogue. Remember, your body believes what you tell it. So, if you are telling yourself that things aren't working out for you, you are reinforcing your belief. If your body perceives stress, this sends a signal from your brain out to your organs and glands that control your stress hormones, your behaviour, and the decisions you make.

Let's use an example of wanting to bring more love into your life. If you wanted to find new love, this is a wish that you would create consciously. If you believe this can be possible for you, and you are supporting yourself with

---

19 - The RAS is a network of nerves in the brain stem that project anteriorly to the hypothalamus to mediate behaviour, as well as posteriorly to the thalamus and directly to the cortex. The RAS serves as a filter system to notice in our environment more of what we are focused on in our minds, helping us to be more resourceful.

confidence and self-esteem boosting thoughts, then you are creating an alignment with what you want vs. what you believe about yourself and what is possible.

What we believe matters. If our positive beliefs align with our goals, not only is it easier to bring this into our lives, but it also feels good when we can manifest our desires. Alternatively, if we do not believe that we can bring more love into our life, it will be harder to create, and this conflict can lead to stress in the mind and body.

Catch your reactions

You can reimagine what is possible for your mind, body and life. You can change your beliefs, by first recognising them through your reactions, then asking yourself: Are they aligning with what I am trying to create for myself? From there, you can create a new habit by being more observant about what you are saying, feeling and believing. It is eye-opening. Once you see that this is all in your control, it can empower you to create a successful and healthy life, because you deserve this.

It takes anywhere from 2-8 months to create a new habit, according to Lally's study.[20] Have a morning and evening ritual to check in with your mind, thoughts, feelings and body. It is helpful to wear a wristband or any bracelet that can be a prop for you; you can even use an elastic band that you can snap. Wear something you can see to remind you during the day, to catch yourself in those moments when you are reacting or being self-critical. When you get stuck in your head overthinking. Flick it when you catch yourself being negative, when you are assuming worst-case scenarios, or when you are living on autopilot. In those moments, choose a new reaction that is positive, and in alignment with what you are wanting to create.

---

20 - https://www.ncbi.nlm.nih.gov/pmc/articles/PMC3505409/

Train yourself to be more present in the moment, try to let go of the past, and try not to think too much into the future. Right here and right now is what we need to focus on. When we are being conscious and present, we are in our most creative and suggestible state. From this place we can choose a new program, a new narrative, leading to a happier and healthier you.

Meditation and journaling are simple and effective tools to bring yourself back into the moment, promoting a calm mindset and new habits. More about these great tools later.

> ### Hot Tip!
> Our body believes what we tell it. Catch yourself when you are being critical of yourself and choose your thoughts. Flip the thought from negative to positive immediately, then repeat the positive statement:
>
> | | | |
> |---|---|---|
> | *I am not safe* | → | **I have everything that I need** |
> | *I am not heard* | → | **I am heard and acknowledged** |
> | *I am not worthy* | → | **I am enough** |
> | *I am not liked* | → | **I am lovable** |
> | *I am not good enough* | → | **I am magnificent** |
> | *I am not successful* | → | **I have achieved so much** |

Chapter 8
The Art of Bending Like Bamboo

When we Bend Like Bamboo, we are anchored just like a bamboo tree.

When we discover our inner anchor, this allows us to be more flexible and resilient. We adapt to change, we get out of our comfort zone, we are at our best.

When we Bend Like Bamboo, we encompass resilience and flexibility in our mind, body and life. We discover our inner anchor, which allows us to be more grounded and connected.

To Bend Like Bamboo is to be flexible and adaptable in times of change. It is the ability to adapt and see our situation with fresh eyes. It is the ability to reimagine what can be possible in our minds, bodies and lives. It is the ability to see our obstacles as opportunities from a higher perspective. It is the ability to lean into uncertainty with confidence. It is the ability to get out of our comfort zone to grow.

When we are tired, stressed and anxious we tend to overthink the future, and become stuck in the past, living in autopilot. This impacts our ability to be at our best, at home, at work and within our relationships.

It is a mindset, and when you are stressed, tired and feel disengaged, you may believe there is no way out. The truth is that right now you have no idea how adaptable you are.

We can let go of rigidity and stress, we become more flexible. Flexibility in our mindset impacts everything that matters: our body's ability to repair, how happy and resilient we are, and how connected we can be. Anchored and flexible, we can change our mind about old stories, we can let go of what is old and redundant.

When we are flexible, we are more able to adapt and see our situation with fresh eyes and a higher perspective; we can think in new and innovative directions. Anchored and flexible, when the wind comes in life we are prepared, we believe in our ability to keep going and to overcome. As resilience increases, we can lean into uncertainty with confidence, getting out of our comfort zone to where we will grow. On my journey, I have learned that this can be the best environment to maximise performance and the body's ability to repair.

It is an elevated mindset that is more malleable and adaptable, where we can access more elevated emotions, such as joy, compassion, forgiveness and courage. Letting go of lower and denser emotions such as guilt, shame, anger and worry. When we are in this more flexible state, we are more adaptable. We can optimise creativity, performance and our wellbeing.

Bending with change

There will be moments when you'll surprise yourself by what is possible, it is from here you'll begin to see possibility everywhere.

Amanda Campbell

Change happens every day of our lives, but sometimes life brings bigger changes like divorce, death or illness.

When we are stressed, we become more rigid and close-minded, and this impacts on our health, happiness and how we show up in the world. We can be in our heads, overthinking, stuck in the past or overanalysing the future. But when we are calmer and more present, we are in our most creative state and in the best environment to promote repair.[21]

Setbacks are designed to move us; we are supposed to feel uncomfortable when we experience change. When we feel stretched from a space of rigidity within ourselves, change can be perceived as a setback. Instead, could we see our setbacks as detours to the next destination we are ready for? This perspective can reduce suffering, anxiety and a loss of energy, allowing us to maintain a positive and calmer state, that maximises energy.

---

[21] - Bruce H. Lipton, Ph.D., cell biologist and lecturer, is an internationally recognised leader in bridging science and spirit. Bruce was on the faculty of the University of Wisconsin's School of Medicine and later performed groundbreaking stem cell research at Stanford Medical School. His pioneering research on cloned human stem cells presaged today's revolutionary new field of epigenetics. He is the bestselling author of *The Biology of Belief* and *The Honeymoon Effect* and discusses survival vs. growth and repair pathways.

When we can see life from a higher perspective, we are able to connect the dots and understand that a change in direction is a path guiding us to where we need to go. Change is difficult and we are tempted to resist it. But if we train ourselves to be more flexible, less reactive and more open to possibility, we can better master change.

In a fast-paced, modern world filled with stress and excessive external stimulation, we can become rigid and closed, and it feels like we must just get through the day. We can forget to question our thoughts and feelings, and we can forget what meaning we are placing on our circumstances, what we are believing about ourselves, and therefore what can be possible in our lives.

There is a better way. I believe the first point of action is to give ourselves the best environment to be open to change. If flexibility builds resilience, which can promote repair, could a flexible mindset allow us to feel healthier and happier? When we are feeling happy, healthy and flexible, we are more inclined to push ourselves out of our comfort zone, face our fears and be open to change.

Dealing with change

From my personal experience and from observations when working with clients, what seems to hold many of us back from making the shifts required is that we are afraid of the chaos. Chaos can be from past trauma, so we can convince ourselves that if we lean into uncertainty and take a risk, we may fall into difficult times of chaos all over again. Because it can be safer to think of worst-case scenarios, we need to consciously focus on the positive, to make it possible for us to change our minds and lean in.

The trick is to give yourself the best environment to shift an alarmed state, so your brain can stop perceiving threat and danger, letting go of shock and stress, helping you to feel calm and resilient. In this positive mindset, you can experience your nervous system literally putting the brakes on; you have a deeper connection to your gut instinct and are guided to knowing what to do. You will open your mind to new possibilities and think in innovative new directions, professionally and personally.

Once you know what direction you are taking, it is easier to know the next step. Focus on what you want and on the joy that this new direction will bring you. Imagine it, feel it, and embody the mindset you want to be in; feel the joy as if you have it already. I highly recommend processing your emotions and thoughts, helping to wash and empty the mind with daily journaling and meditation, which we will explore in later chapters.

What we believe is what matters. Can you find the courage to believe that when you make this change, when you stare into the abyss of uncertainty, that things will go well for you? To make things happen for yourself, can you align your desire with what you believe can be possible? Align your mind and body with your gut instinct, spirit and guidance. Then as you go through the change, things will start to appear more effortless for you. Try not to focus on negative scenarios in your mind; focus only on how exciting the new direction will be, and on the joy that is coming your way.

My model of change

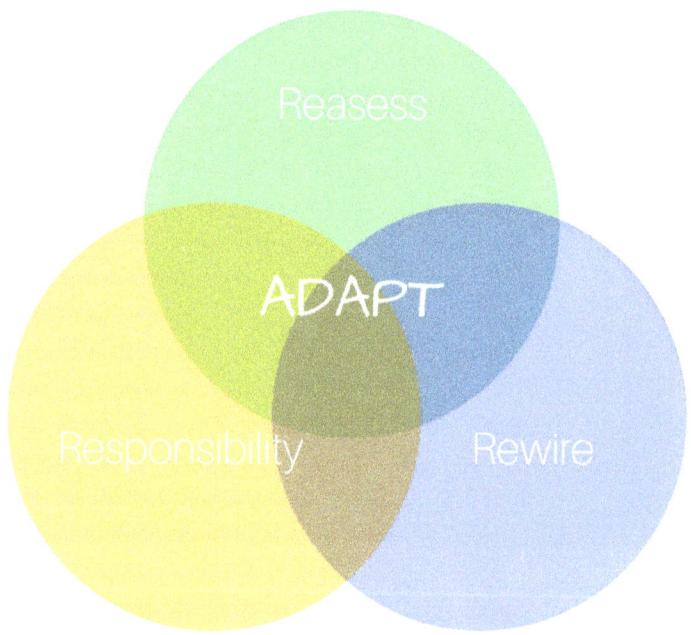

My model of change involves 3 stages:

1. **Reassess with awareness.** Awareness is the greatest agent for change. First, we need to be aware of what is blocking us. We do a great job of burying our inner conflicts, then when difficult emotions arise and they are too painful, we suppress them to cope. Over time, we can lose touch with how we really feel, who we really are, and what we really want in our lives. Becoming aware of our inner conflict and understanding the cause of what is holding us back can empower us to transform and heal.

2. **Responsibility.** When we are aware, we can take responsibility for our mindset, perceptions, health and the results in our life. We are responsible for our own state, and we get to choose our reactions. We can change our mind about what we are believing about ourselves or our situation. Taking responsibility is empowering, and when we take our power back, we can see our circumstances through fresh eyes. Taking more responsibility leads to flexibility, new ideas, beliefs, behaviours and habits, as well as seeing obstacles as opportunities.

3. **Rewire the brain.** When empowered with understanding and the clarity of a path forward, we can take steps to rewire our brain. It takes a minimum 21–66 days to create a new habit[22], so consistency is key. Neurones that fire together, wire together. When we learn to focus on what we want, we feel more positive and we open to possibility, promoting adaptability and resilience.

Reassess with awareness

Reassessing our behaviour requires flexibility. We can get so stuck in our stories, many of them stressful, old and redundant, triggering negative thoughts, habits and sabotage. For this reason, I find it productive to consciously reassess what I am thinking, feeling and believing on a regular basis. Bringing awareness into our day, especially in the mornings, can be the catalyst for transformation. By simply noticing our reactions, we can bring more awareness into our lives.

---

22 - On average, it takes more than 2 months before a new behaviour becomes automatic – 66 days to be exact. And how long it takes a new habit to form can vary widely, depending on the behaviour, the person and the circumstances. Phillippa Lally is a health psychology researcher at University College London. In a study published in the European Journal of Social Psychology, Lally and her research team decided to figure out just how long it actually takes to form a habit. In Lally's study, it took anywhere from 18 days to 254 days for people to form a new habit. https://www.ncbi.nlm.nih.gov/pmc/articles/PMC3505409/

Our reactions are a mirror image of what we believe. If what we believe is what really matters, could being more aware of any negative beliefs be the link to untangling what is causing us stress? Can you get out of your story, just for a moment, and view your life as an observer, from a bird's eye perspective?

Catch your reactions. When you find yourself focused on negative, worst-case scenarios and what you don't want, practise bringing your awareness back into the moment. When you are in your head, overthinking the past or overanalysing the future, catch yourself and bring yourself back into the moment.

I use a prop to do this, because I am human and I can forget. A wristband works well: I have created *Bend Like Bamboo* wristbands for my clients that help them to be present and to remember what they are working on. They have mantras on them like 'I am enough' and when I see it on my wrist, I remember to catch myself. When we are more aware of what is blocking us, what we are suppressing, and usually what we have been avoiding for a while, we can take responsibility to make the required changes to transform this within ourselves. We can also elevate our mindset and energy morning and evening with journaling, meditation, hydration, nutrition and movement.

Responsibility

When we are aware of what is blocking us, we can begin to take responsibility to change it. When we know why we do what we do, we can find love and compassion to empower ourselves to adapt and grow. We can untangle years of sabotage and move towards a life filled with love and success. There are many ways to take responsibility; there is an opportunity to do so with every choice that we make. Every time we think or speak, we can choose who we want to be and how we will react.

Once we are aware of what is blocking us or holding us back, we can see our situation with new eyes and with greater understanding. Then we can take responsibility for where we are. We can apply new meaning to our situation, and therefore feel differently.

How we feel is so important; when we feel good, we can be more flexible and open to change. We can be kinder and more compassionate towards another person's point of view. We can grow and learn; we can problem-solve faster. Taking full responsibility for every aspect of our life is empowering, because it allows us to step into our power. It is from this place we will embrace the lessons and walk a new unpaved path, with courage and excitement. We embark on a journey filled with greater meaning and purpose, more nourishing for our mind, body and spirit.

Rewire the brain

When we have the courage to rise from a fall, we are ready to face our shadows and fears. Bringing awareness to our inner resistance helps us to take responsibility. With this mindset, we can begin to rewire our brains and integrate a new way of being. We can become a whole new version of ourselves.

After we go through trying times, a new person emerges at the other end. Our thinking, our beliefs and our vocabulary are literally transformed. We are not the same as we were before. As a result, the way we experience stress and how we receive joy shifts. As a result of that, a new biochemistry can fire. I believe that this is how we can begin to experience a new mind, body and life.

As we step into this new version of ourselves, a part of us must die off, like a butterfly emerging from its cocoon. When we go through a transformation, we instinctively know that we are in the dark and that we must be still during this time. It's tempting to pierce the wall – it's dark and we don't know what is going to happen next. But the day will come when it's time to spread our wings and fly.

We can rewire our brain with repetition, daily consistency is key. I love doing something that scares me every day, as I am building resilience in my mindset, getting out of my comfort zone. When this becomes familiar for you, you can feel unstoppable!

We can rewire our brain to be open to new habits, routines and possibilities. We create stories to make sense of things. Have you noticed that some of the stories you've created are true, but sometimes they're based on assumed facts and perceptions or limiting beliefs?

Catch yourself when you go into autopilot, by using a wristband or any prop that reminds you to stop yourself in the moment. I reset my reaction by asking myself: Is this thought true? Am I feeling stressed about what is going on right now? Or is my current situation triggering something stressful from the past?

Dr. Joe Dispenza is a bestselling author, expert from *What the BLEEP Do We Know!?*, chiropractic doctor and famous lecturer on neuroscience and quantum physics. He explains that the more you focus on what you want, the less synapses will fire to the old memories that make you focus on the negative.[23] Could this be a way for us to rewire how our brain fires? When we learn to focus consistently on what we want, we begin to feel safer and calmer, letting go of fear and stress. Synapses that used to fire to old fearful memories will stop firing, rewiring to new and more positive pathways.

I recommend starting with smaller changes; they will translate into bigger ones. For example, brush your teeth with a different hand; dry yourself differently when you get out of the shower; go to new places on your lunch break. Most of all, seek joy in your life again. In my experience

---

23 - https://drjoedispenza.com/

and from seeing clients at my practice, I have observed the power of shifting into an elevated mindset, helping us to be more open to joy and receiving. Our ability to see opportunities for growth from our adversities allows us to accept and forgive them, joyfully. We can heal any inner conflict within us, walk away from sabotaging cycles in our lives, and embrace change with flexibility and resilience. I believe that our ability to let more joy in can saturate every cell of our being, healing us in ways we are yet to understand.

How I learned to Bend Like Bamboo

I had to learn this the hard way. When I was paralysed, it was terrifying and I felt out of control. All I wanted was for it to go away. But once I stopped using most of my energy resisting and focusing on what I didn't want, I began to swim downstream instead of up. I had to embrace the inevitable, to fall into the black abyss of the unknown. As a result, I had more energy and inspiration to optimise my mind, my health and situation.

Life is always about continual adjustment. Just like a plane flying. It doesn't follow a direct, straight path to get to its destination, it is constantly adjusting to stay on course. If we can alter the way we feel about change, we can welcome it as an important process of life.

For me, it was only when I had no choice but to surrender that I was able to drop the fear, because I wanted to overcome the MS symptoms that were literally paralysing me. I embraced what was happening to my body, and I let go of wanting to have complete control. I had no choice other than to say to myself, 'Well, this is happening. I cannot control it, so bring it on!' And that attitude had more surrender to it, more flow. Ironically, tackling my fears head-on was nowhere near as hard as I thought it would be. And as a result, I was happier and became more connected to myself, my mind and my body. The most magical part of all was that I began to heal faster than I ever could have imagined was possible.

The concept of Bending Like Bamboo was birthed as I went on a journey to learn how to give my mind and body the best environment to be open for repair and transformation. The same formula has helped me to navigate change in my life and overcome some big curve balls with a more resilient mindset.

On my journey I discovered that the pillars of health (mind, body, food and connection) were key. Connecting a happy mind with a happy body, while nourishing it with happy food, promoted a reconnection for me that changed my life.

My Story in a Snapshot

I stand here today against all odds and I'd love the share my story with you about how I learned to Bend Like Bamboo.

When I was young, I was always a motivated, happy and driven girl. My twin sister Nicole and I were both lucky to attend schools that not only offered academics, but also sports and music. We had a passion for music, so much so we learned flute, violin, piano and trained in singing and dance. We become obsessed, leading us to pursue a career in music where we sang and wrote our own music. We were living the dream.

At age 19, we were studying music theatre and dance full time; this was the year I first experienced pins and needles down the left-hand side of my face and fingertips. I went to my local GP who then ordered an MRI. They found one lesion on my brain, but there was no diagnosis. Eventually it all resolved, and I just got on with my life.

I fell into the fashion industry, a career I loved throughout my 20s. At age 24, my symptoms came back. But this time, the numbness progressed to weakness. Another MRI showed 2 new lesions in my brain, and I was diagnosed with MS. From that moment on, everything just stopped. Feeling stressed and uncertain about my future, I began to focus on what I didn't want and what I feared. That I might end up disabled, bedridden or worse. So, I went out later, I worked harder, and disconnected more and more from the inner conflict that was brewing in my body. Externally I was still driven I worked hard with a smile on my face. But on the inside, I was terrified and wanted to disconnect from the fear and pain.

MS is a disease of the central nervous system, the brain, optic nerves and the spinal cord. When you have MS, your body believes that it needs to attack the myelin that protects all our nerves. It is an incorrect signal that we are yet to understand. Picture a phone charger, the white plastic is the myelin that protect all our nerves (the wires) on the inside. The myelin acts as a conductor allowing electrical impulses to fire out to our body. Therefore, symptoms can include blindness, paralysis, inability to swallow, digestive issues, cognitive changes, heat sensitivity and nerve pain.

Five years later, living in fear, my inner conflict brewed. I began to believe that I wasn't going to be okay. I started to believe that I would not be able to achieve all the things I wanted for my life, professionally and personally. The symptoms came back at age 29, and I had the biggest relapse of my life. Over a slow cruel 10 days, the entire left-hand side of my body become completely paralysed. My face dropped, my left arm twisted, my hip, leg and foot just completely stopped working on the left side of my body. I lost the ability to walk, wash and feed myself, and I simply couldn't get dressed without help. I lost my financial independence, my ability to work, and my life as I knew it. It had to completely stop and reset.

In one of my first rehab sessions, I remember doing an exercise the physio gave me of trying to make just my fingers open and close. I had tears running down my face, because it was so hard. I knew that in that moment, I had a choice. I could either give up … or … I had to change my mind about what I believed could be possible, to get different results.

Something shifted within me. Like a woman on a mission, I was first in at physio and last to leave. One day my toe moved for the first time, out of the blue. It was in that moment I found hope and as a result, I started to channel my energy differently. With hope and more belief of what could be possible, I began to focus on what I wanted, rather than what I didn't want.

It is amazing what happens inside of yourself when you have no choice but to succeed. They said that I may never walk again, and I was 29 years old. It was the hardest, darkest time of my life. If you light a candle in a well-lit room, you don't so much notice the light. But when everything becomes dark, that is when you can find your own light, and what you are truly made of.

I walked and ran within 6 weeks. Deemed a rapid recovery, I began to study and research how I recovered when I wasn't 'supposed to'. I immersed myself into understanding the mind-body connection, the art of repair and transformation.

What I learned was that what we believe is really important. Feeling more relaxed and flexible, we can let go of control and certainty, and the inner resistance that is fuelling a stress response. We surrender into a flow state that reconnects us. This can become the best environment we can give the mind and body to let go of stress and negativity, shifting into positivity and an environment that can promote repair.

I now understand that setbacks are designed to move us. We are supposed to feel uncomfortable, so that we move towards a new direction that is in fact our path. Otherwise, we would stay in the comfort of where we are! This requires getting out of our comfort zone. I had to master making the unfamiliar familiar, and began to make the familiar (bad habits, negative behaviour) unfamiliar.

In my personal experience and now as a trained Sports Kinesiologist, I am astounded by the mind-body connection and have been able to identify patterns. When we are stressed, the subconscious and old fear-based programs dominate, and we are not our best selves. When we are stressed, we have a more closed and rigid mindset. When we are more relaxed and present, we feel more resilient, we believe in ourselves, and transformation is possible.

Working hard to grow my business, I had to be on top of my game to perform. I learned that the power of flexibility that had helped me to promote repair in my mind and body, also applied to promoting optimal performance when at work. A flexible mindset helps us to relax and destress. With a more elevated mindset we are more confident and solution-focused.

When we are managing stress and anchoring within ourselves, this becomes integrated through our relationships and work culture. Our elevated and positive state becomes contagious, as we are all so connected.

A happy mind is connected to a happy body while we are nourishing it with happy foods. When we eat better, we feel better. When we feel like a leader, we think and act like a leader too.

What is multiple sclerosis?

Multiple sclerosis (MS) is a chronic disease of the central nervous system and is most common among Australians between 20 and 50 years of age, with Victorians rated the highest of those diagnosed. Although MS can be progressive and unpredictable, it is not contagious.

MS occurs when the protective sheath (myelin) around the nerve fibres in the brain and spinal cord becomes damaged from a confused message in the immune response to attack it. When the protective myelin becomes damaged, it causes random patches called plaques or lesions. These patches distort and interrupt the messages sent along the nerves. 'Sclerosis' means 'scarring' and the disease is labelled 'multiple' because the damage usually occurs at several points.

Symptoms of MS can include:

- motor control: muscular spasms, weakness, loss of coordination, loss of balance, loss of arm and leg function, paralysis
- neurological: vertigo, pins and needles, visual disturbances, blindness
- neuropsychological: memory loss, cognitive changes, anxiety, depression
- organ stress: bladder urgency/frequency, constipation, digestive issues
- fatigue
- heat sensitivity and nerve pain

I mentioned earlier in my story that a phone charger is a great analogy of what can happen to your central nervous system (CNS) when you have MS. The 'white plastic' represents the myelin that protects the nerves, allowing electrical impulses to fire out from your brain and spine to your muscles, nerves, organs and the systems of the body. When you have an attack of MS, your body believes the myelin is foreign and so it is attacked. This causes damage to the 'white plastic' that represents the insular coating of the myelin, which has the job of protecting the nerves in your brain, spine, eyes and central nervous system.

The disease is unpredictable and at times progressive. Messages that are sent along the myelin become distorted, which leads to symptoms that can be neurological, psychological and physical.

There are many different health effects from this disease and no two people share the same symptoms. The cause of MS is unknown and as yet there is no cure. However, treatments are available to slow down the course of the disease. Some people live with a very benign case and luckily do not progress into disability. We still do not understand why this happens and why some people go the other way.

MS Fast Facts

- Globally, an estimated 2,800,000 people have MS.
- Approximately 33,000 Australians have been diagnosed.
- 3 out of 4 people that are diagnosed are women.
- 4 people a week are diagnosed in Australia; 200 a week in USA.
- Most are diagnosed between the ages of 20 and 50.

Autoimmune diseases

- There are over 80 different autoimmune conditions. Some are well known, such as type 1 diabetes, multiple sclerosis, lupus, rheumatoid arthritis, alopecia, celiac disease and psoriasis, while others are rare and difficult to diagnose.

- With unusual autoimmune diseases, patients may suffer for years before getting a proper diagnosis. Most of these diseases have no cure. Some require lifelong treatment to ease symptoms.

- Each autoimmune condition attacks a different part of the body.

- Localised autoimmune disorders affect one part of the body e.g., MS affects the central nervous system.

- Systemic autoimmune disorders affect more than one part of the body e.g., rheumatoid arthritis affects the joints and sometimes the skin, lungs and eyes.

- Women tend to be more commonly affected by autoimmune conditions.

- Approximately 1 in 20 people are affected by autoimmune disorders.

- Autoimmune conditions range widely in severity and no two cases are the same.

- Autoimmune conditions can go undiagnosed for years; some cases show no obvious symptoms.[24]

---

24 - https://www.niehs.nih.gov/health/topics/conditions/autoimmune/index.cfm

Chapter 9
The Power of Kinesiology

When I was 31 years old, I changed my career from the fashion industry after experiencing enormous change in my life. I was rebuilding my mind, body and life, after recovering from a MS attack that paralysed me. A kinesiologist and physiotherapist helped me to walk again, so I was inspired to go back to school to study Sports Kinesiology. I learned about Chinese medicine concepts of the mind-body connection, anatomy and physiology. My studies explored the body's connection structurally, biochemically, emotionally and electromagnetically. This was the first time I had understood the body in such an integrated way, rather than seeing it in isolation. I discovered that we don't think or function in isolation; there are many moving dynamic parts, all connected in a very powerful way that we are yet to fully understand.

Kinesiology understands that the muscles are connected to the brain via the nervous system. Kinesiologists use the muscles to understand the health and state of our organs and systems of the body. When tested, the integrity of our muscles gives the practitioner feedback and an insight into the mind-body connection and any imbalances that need to be assessed.

Taking a wholistic approach helps a trained practitioner to find the cause of a physical, emotional, biochemical or energetic imbalance, as there are often many moving parts to the equation, along with subconscious programs to consider. I find kinesiology to be effective for both physical and emotional disorders. Some examples are relief from symptoms of disease, fertility issues, addiction, menopause, anxiety, worry and stress, pain, inflammation, allergies, injuries, weight loss and inflammation.

Kinesiology is effective for optimising performance and learning, identifying our barriers to achieving our goals, and is one of the most powerful modalities that I have ever experienced. In every session, I feel like I have returned back to myself; I experience an alignment of my mind, body and spirit. I feel lighter, clearer and more relaxed. I am better able to manage stress and take on life's challenges with a positive and resilient mindset.

Our thinking and beliefs matter, because our muscles connect into the subconscious brain unlocking habits, behaviours and beliefs that may be holding us back, kinesiology is a helpful tool to access these subconscious programs that impact our wellbeing and how we show up in the world. For example, failure to work through any of the various emotions associated with mourning and loss can result in prolonged depression and prolonged states of denial. Chronic guilt or the refusal to work through the emotions associated with loss can result in delayed grief reaction and physical disease. The suppressed energy of relinquished emotions re-emerges through the body's endocrine and nervous systems as an energetic imbalance, which impairs the flow of life energy through the body's acupuncture meridians. This can result in pathological changes to various organs. It is a well-known fact that the death rate of the bereaved is much higher than that of the general population, especially in the first year or two following the death of a spouse.

David Hawkins discusses the effects of suppressed and repressed feelings in his life-changing book, *Letting Go*.[25] He explains that stress-precipitating factors are

---

25 - https://www.veritaspub.com/author/David-R-Hawkins

responsible for most emotional and physical illnesses. There is an emotional-psychological component in all disease and, because of this, it can be possible to reverse the disease process by removing the internal stress factors. This accounts for the many recoveries, reported daily, from serious and potentially fatal illnesses using emotional-spiritual techniques.

Many cures take place after all medical methods have failed. At the stage when there is 'nothing else we can do', patients seek and accept the true basic nature and reason for their illness. They are forced to find the answers within. Acknowledging and letting go of suppressed feelings reduces a person's personal stress proneness, thereby lowering their vulnerability to stress-related problems and illnesses. Most people who learn and practise a 'letting go' technique notice a progressive improvement in physical health and vitality.

Kinesiologists navigate the mind and body using the Chinese Medicine Five Elements that connect the muscles to meridians and organs. To this day, the efficacy of it blows my mind! Learning the emotional links to physical ailments, inflammation and disease assists me to get to the root cause of issues that I could not resolve before. It was such a game changer for my life and my health, and I am so grateful I found this modality.

In Eastern medicine, the body is defined by an elaborate array of energy pathways called meridians. In the Chinese physiological chart of the human body, these energy networks resemble electronic wiring. Using aids like acupuncture needles and muscle testing, Chinese physicians test their patients' energy circuits in the same way that electrical engineers 'troubleshoot' a printed circuit board, searching for electrical 'pathologies'.

Our muscles are connected to our brain via our nervous system, and these muscles form groups that are connected to the organs in our bodies. Using the muscles as a feedback tool, kinesiologists access subconscious programs and emotional states that are often out of conscious awareness. Kinesiologists assess the anatomy as a whole, rather than in isolated elements, to look for the cause of what is blocking or sabotaging progress, whether structural, biochemical, emotional or electromagnetic.

To create real change, we need to target the subconscious pathways in the brain that are in charge of approximately 95% of our biochemical processes and reactions. It is not enough to just consciously wish for a change – if only it were that simple! Luckily, kinesiology communicates directly with the subconscious brain, via the muscles and meridians, so much more comes to light and it opens the doorway for transformation and repair.

Our body works as a whole and is so connected, knowing how to navigate its multiple layers helps tremendously with trouble shooting to get to the cause of stress. When we break down the many moving parts into smaller pieces, so much information is revealed. This what inspired me to study Sports Kinesiology.

Qi Flow

Kinesiology is often described as working with a mysterious energy called Qi, that circulates through metaphysical meridians in the body.

When the flow of Qi through our meridians becomes blocked, illness results. The purpose of Kinesiology (and other energetic therapies) is to promote the proper flow of Qi through the meridians, thus restoring health and wellbeing.

In the human body Qi is perceived to flow as 'energy' along the meridian, providing life force, which gives vitality and harmony to the body's overall functions. Within each person, Qi warms the body, retains the body's fluids and organs, fuels the transformation of food into other substances such as Xue (blood), and protects the body from disease.

We can create, preserve, or deplete our Qi by the air we breathe, the food we eat, and the way we consciously balance our body, mind and spirit. Qi therefore not only denotes one's energy flow, but also denotes one's individual energy patterns."[26]

---

26 - https://damianbrown.com.au/

Acupuncture studies

Regarding acupuncture in general, there are a wealth of studies on needle acupuncture. Acupuncture has been shown to be an effective modality across a range of conditions. Its mechanisms of action have been well demonstrated, and we are continuing to discover more about how it works.

Perhaps the best scientific review demonstrating the effectiveness of acupuncture is the meta-analysis by Vickers et al. in 2012. This was a review of individual patient data for nearly 18,000 patients from 29 randomised control trials and clearly showed that acupuncture was effective for pain relief in chronic headache, neck and back pain, shoulder pain and osteoarthritis, to a high degree of significance statistically.[27] For more information on studies of acupuncture, I highly recommend Dr Ballard's book, *Laser Acupuncture.* He specialises in medical acupuncture treatment using laser acupuncture.

My first experience of kinesiology was when I was quite young, thanks to my parents being open to an East meets West approach for our health. May Clarke was one of the first Kinesiologists I had a session with. In some of my first sessions I just cried the whole time, releasing in a positive way; it felt like I was releasing stored emotions that I didn't even know had become stagnant in my body. The sessions felt like I was having a conversation with someone who knew everything about me: physically, biochemically,

---

27 - *Laser Acupuncture,* by Dr. Ralph Ballard

emotionally, as well as my purpose and life path. I was blown away at the accuracy with which the practitioner, whom I had never met before, could gather information and understand me in such accurate detail.

I have had the honour of working with many kinesiologists. Dr. Michael Bay was an applied kinesiologist who helped me to understand kinesiology and its ability to help the body physically, while I was recovering from paralysis. Michael's sessions had such an impact on me. There is another kinesiologist that has also been an incredible part of my healing journey and also in my career as a Sports Kinesiologist. Damian Brown ND, B.Ed.[28] is a leading kinesiologist, naturopath and nutritionist, with a focus on evidence-based practice and the art of healing. Damian has been studying, practising and teaching natural medicine for more than 15 years. We met when kinesiologist Jacque Mooney[29] invited Dr. Charles Krebs to Australia to teach kinesiology masterclasses. Dr. Krebs is a research scientist, university lecturer and the founder of the Learning Enhancement Acupressure Program (LEAP)[30]. He is also the author of *Energetic Kinesiology* and arguably the best kinesiologist in the world, because of his knowledge and background in science and the brain.

We worked on professional athletes together, and he taught us a form of advanced kinesiology; in particular, how to apply brain integration structurally to sports injury and performance. He also taught me how to work with the bladder organ, to treat symptoms of frequency and urgency, a common MS symptom. This has been one of my MS symptoms and rectifying it was a life-changing experience that has helped me profoundly.

---

28 - https://damianbrown.com.au/
29 - https://simplythebrain.com/
30 - https://www.i-leap.org/

Damian and I were upskilling in our own studies and decided to take his class. Since then, I have also studied Damian's masterclasses in kinesiology and nutrition, the thyroid, reproductive, adrenal and immune systems. I still see Damian regularly for my own kinesiology treatments, and he has become a trusted colleague and friend. He guided me through a Kundalini awakening[31] in one of our sessions. For me, that was amazing and a catalyst for deep change and transformation in my life. It was such a surreal and life-changing experience, feeling a wave of energy spiral up my spine. My arms opened involuntarily, and my body waved like a mermaid. I felt a profound sense of love and a grounding and elevation like never before. It was a sacred experience that has opened my insight, intuition and mind in many ways. I now experience a deeper connection to my intuition when I am working on clients. This opening has helped me to open my heart and feel more compassion with my clients and for myself.

In 2020, we started a podcast called *Connect with Damian and Amanda*, sharing interesting and inspiring topics that open possibilities for health, healing and transformation. This podcast can be found on my website.[32]

Kinesiology is one of the biggest gifts that has come into my life. It is a powerful modality that has helped me get to the bottom of my inner conflict. It helps me to navigate life, gets to the bottom of mental and physical ailments, and it brings me guidance and clarity. Kinesiology helps me to connect all the dots, making sense of the many moving parts that make up the mind and body that are physical, mental, emotional, intuitive, intellectual, biochemical, spiritual and energetic.

---

31 - A Kundalini awakening is a form of energetic healing that causes us to transform on mental, emotional and spiritual levels. Kundalini is a form of divine feminine energy located at the base of the spine, in the maladhara.

32 - https://www.amandacampbell.com.au/podcasts

When I studied kinesiology, it was like I sat down at a piano and could play straightaway. I just got it and could see how I could use my ability to feel energy in a way that could move and unblock imbalances. I learned to use the technique as a tool to heal my own imbalances. The results were so outstanding that I decided to dedicate my life to helping others do the same.

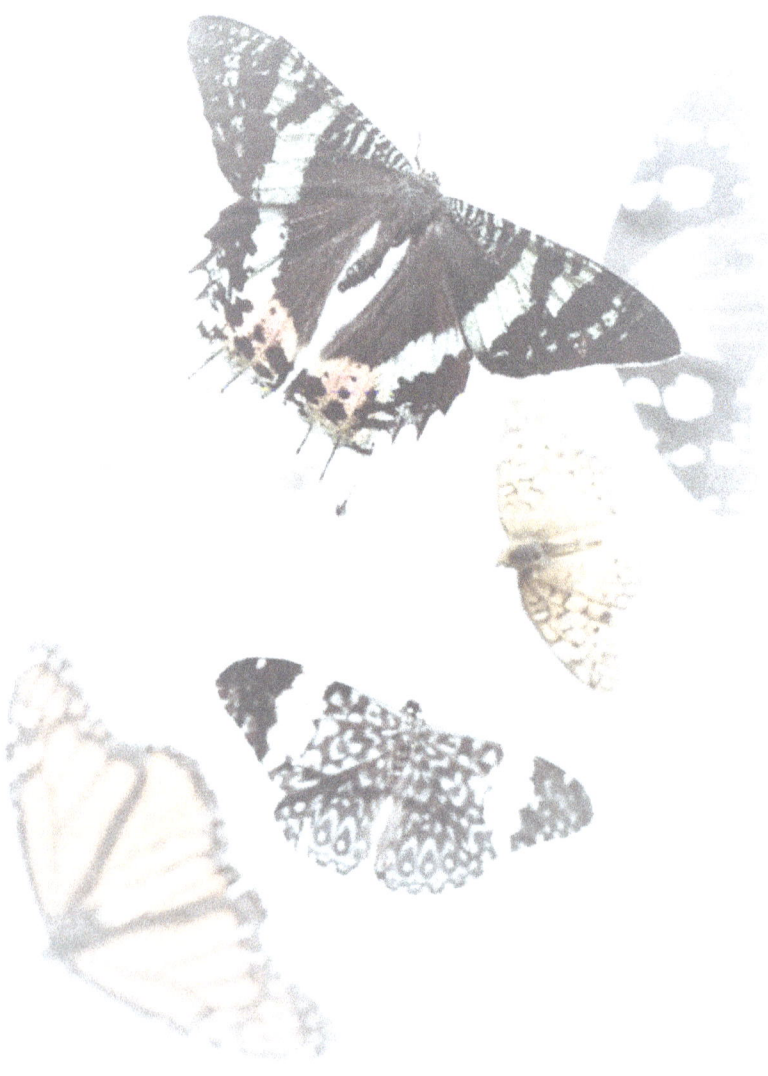

Chapter 10
The Bend Like Bamboo Program

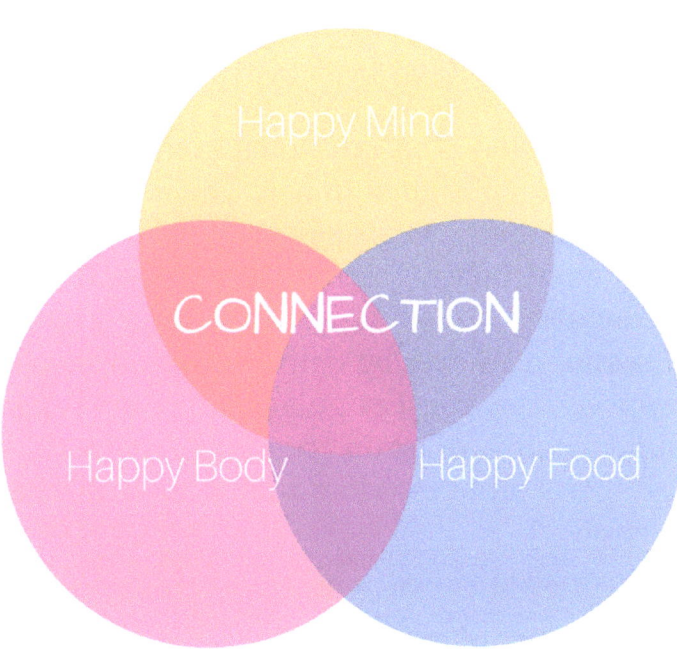

The Bend Like Bamboo program combines the 4 pillars of health of mind, body, food and connection. It also includes tools of meditation and journaling, to build a flexible mindset and resilient attitude. The program is divided into 6 sessions that can be done online, live virtually or in person.

The power of self-belief and resilience

The resilience lesson is an introduction into the Bend Like Bamboo program, designed to help you adapt and master change with flexibility. In a kinesiology session, we explore your goals, your beliefs, mental and physical symptoms and any diagnosis.

This session can also be delivered as an inspirational keynote speech (my most popular one) or an in-person or virtual interactive workshop for people at work, kids at school or sports athletes. More information can be found on my website.[33]

The topics covered are:

- Amanda's story of recovery
- The power of self-belief and resilience
- The art of Bending Like Bamboo and flexibility
- How to adapt to change
- Transforming obstacles into opportunities
- A resilience formula

---

33 - www.bendlikebamboo.com

Goal setting

This session revolves around asking yourself 6 questions:

1. What is a fear I want to overcome?
2. What is my desire or goal?
3. Do I feel inner resistance about it?
4. Do I believe in myself?
5. Do I believe in what can be possible?
6. How do I sabotage myself?

Exercise: *Goal setting*

This exercise will help you explore what you believe about yourself and whether you believe it can be possible for you.

Have a little think and decide on the most important goal in your life right now. Take a blank sheet of paper and write this goal down on the top left corner of your page. For example, your goal might be: *I want to attract love into my life*. Don't overthink it; just write down something that comes to mind straight from your heart.

Now next to that goal, on the top right of the page, write down the positive beliefs you have about yourself, your worth, your ability to achieve it, and what you believe can be possible for you. For example, if your goal is to receive more love this may be: *I'm kind and loving; I have empathy; I have an open heart and I am ready to receive love in my life*.

Further down the page, underneath the positive beliefs, write down any negative beliefs or fears you might have about your ability to achieve your goal or why it is not possible for you. For example, that might be: *Relationships never last; I am not lovable enough OR I do not believe this will happen for me OR I do not know how to create this for myself OR I do not know what is right for me*.

Which beliefs do your goals align more closely with? The positive ones? Or are there more negative beliefs that conflict with your goal? I call this the 'inner conflict'. Discovering your inner conflict is the most important thing you can do for yourself. It can lead you to the emotional cause of stress, inflammation, pain, disease, insomnia and sabotage. My goal is to help you to understand what is behind the resistance you feel, when your goals are not aligned with what you believe about yourself and what can be possible for you. This exercise can help you to discover what is making you fatigued and stressed, impacting your health.

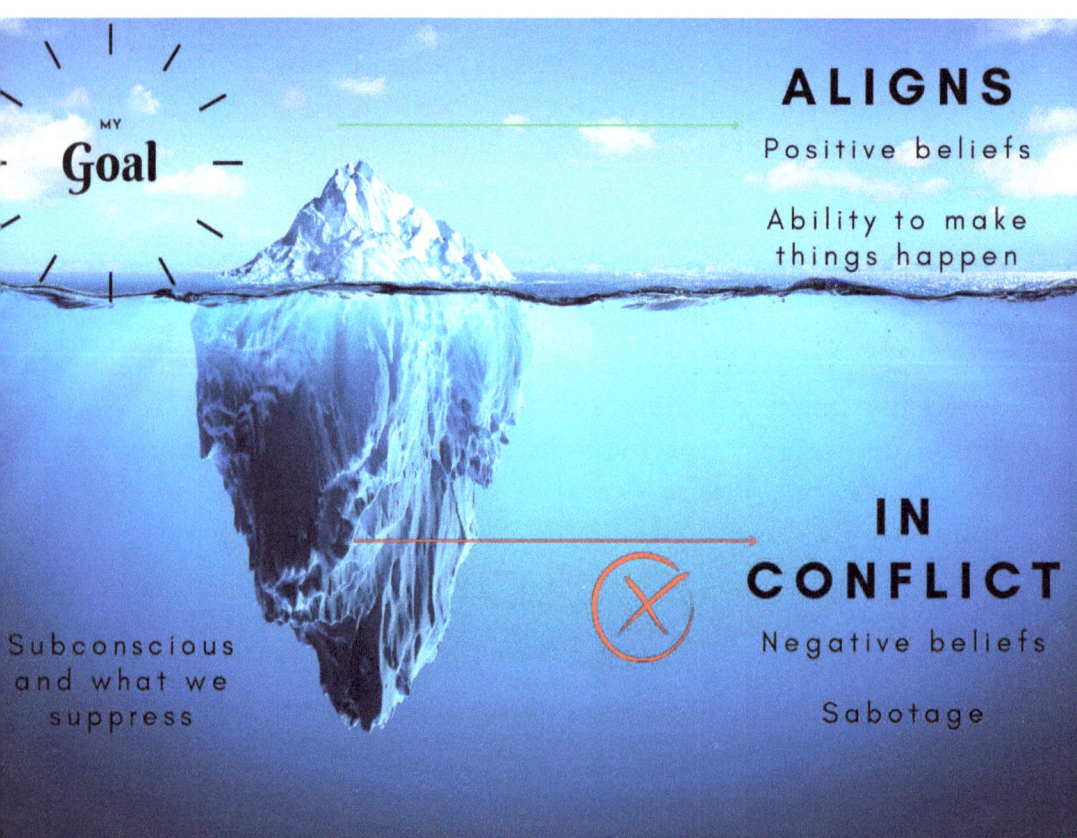

The inner conflict vs. alignment of goals and positive beliefs

It is important to ask yourself: Are any of these beliefs or old stories true? Why do I have these beliefs? When did they start? Are they old and redundant now? Are they serving me? Are they making me feel stressed or making me feel good? How does it serve me to stay in this negative pattern? Am I punishing myself? What do I need to let go of? Can I change my mind about the story I've been telling myself?

When was the last time you questioned your beliefs? It's worth taking time on a regular basis to consciously reconcile your goals with your beliefs. It can be very powerful.

What we believe is what matters. It determines how we react, how we perceive our environment, how stressed we are, and the health of our bodies. If we don't check in and question our beliefs, we can end up living our entire lives from a story that may not be true for us, simply because we have not reviewed old perceptions and let go of the past.

You wash your body every day. How do you wash your mind of negative thoughts, old ideas or redundant habits that are no longer serving your growth? To do this well, we need to get better at letting go.

When we focus on the positive and believe in ourselves, we create more alignment and the resistance can shift. Then it becomes easier to make our goals happen. I believe this is also an optimal environment for healing and change, making a real difference in our lives.

Many of us are living life in a survival pattern, due to the inner conflict of an idea not aligning with what we believe. Often suppressed and unaddressed for a long period of time, this can lead to stressed induced diseases, inflammation, negativity and unhappiness.

When we are stressed, we tend to focus on worst-case scenarios and inevitably what we don't want, because that is the safest way to survive. When what we believe about ourselves conflicts with our goals in life, this misalignment is a stress that sends a survival signal to the body.

However, when our ideas are aligned with what we believe, there is more harmony in the mind and body. I believe that this alignment also connects to the deeper connection we have with the universe, that allows us to manifest and be the creators of our lives.

The good news is that your triggers are a blessing; they are a sign to stop and listen. Listen to your reactions, as they are a mirror image of what you are believing. Within these moments, you can then ask yourself: Is what I believe in conflict with what I want? Can I change my mind about this 'story'? Think of it as an opportunity. When we are faced with an inner conflict, a setback that accompanies fear and a time of stagnation, this can also be a catalyst for growth. When we are faced with bigger changes in life, circumstances or events that require us to dig down deep to find the strength within us that we previously didn't know we had, can be one of the hardest things to overcome.

Looking back at some of the events that I have had to face in my life, what I know now is that it is critical to give our mind and body the best environment to be positive, open-minded, creative and resilient. This allows us to change our mind about what can be possible for us, helping us to become a whole new version of ourselves.

Case study 1

I worked with a guy who wanted to run a marathon. Training was required for fitness and endurance, but he found it hard to find the time to train. Dramas in his life would arise that led him to cancel training. Diving deeper allowed us to discover that he was afraid to fail and so would rather not put himself out there, to try to avoid emotional pain and disappointment.

Case study 2

I worked with a girl who wanted to get a promotion at work, but she was too scared to voice up in meetings, to demonstrate her ability to take on more responsibility. After diving deeper, we came to realise that because she wasn't believing in herself and her possibility and potential, she was unable to stand in her power so that others could believe in her too.

That's how it feels when you want something, but you feel an inner resistance to making it happen for yourself, and how sabotage tends to play out. We must get to the cause of the inner resistance, because what we believe is what matters. Bringing this into her awareness, and adding rituals into her day that helped her to create a more flexible mindset, helped her to change the story she was telling herself. Now she has found her voice and is thriving in her role at work.

So, to recap …

- ✓ Flexibility builds resilience, helping us to optimise our health and performance.

- ✓ When we are stressed, we are more rigid, focused on the negative and are unwell.

- ✓ When we are more present, we can be more creative, solution-focused and happier.

- ✓ What we believe is what matters.

- ✓ A flexible mindset allows us to reimagine what can be possible in our minds, bodies and lives.

Happy mind

Every day you wash your body, but how do you wash your mind? The Happy Mind session is a deeper dive into the power of the mind, and how to promote a flexible mindset that can promote repair and performance. In a kinesiology session, we explore your reactions and your beliefs, and you learn how to rewire your brain to be more positive and resilient. This session can also be delivered as an in-person or virtual presentation, or an interactive workshop for people at work, kids at school or sports athletes. More information can be found on my website.

Flexibility in our mindset impacts on everything that matters:

- our brain's ability to adapt, rewire and repair
- how happy and resilient we are
- how we perform in times of setback
- navigating change effectively
- leading and performing through adversity

How to build a happy mind

With a flexible mindset, we can start to question whether our current habits and behaviours are serving us. Perhaps what we believe is outdated and no longer true. With a flexible mindset, we are more open to the truth. The best environment for flexibility is one where we feel calmer and happier.

We are in charge of our perceptions. Yes, we really are! Our perceptions do stem from motor programs and past experiences, but they are malleable. The brain is much like a computer; it compares current data to past data, to make sense of incoming stimuli. We have a choice in each moment to reassess how we are functioning as a human being, to choose how we think, feel, believe and react. We can change our mind about how we are interpreting our environment by simply learning to question our reactions. It's not always easy, but it's necessary for us to evolve and reach our fullest potential.

If we can master our perceptions and reactions, and can take full responsibility for our lives, life gets really fun! You realise you are the creator of your life with every thought, word and action. The trick is to feel safe enough to change your mind about your beliefs and habits, and to get out of survival mode.

Self-talk and inner dialogue

Our inner dialogue is so important. What we tell ourselves either reinforces old beliefs or builds new ones. Our actions mimic what we believe, so we will inevitably create more of the same around us.

Our body believes what we tell it. Catch yourself when you are being critical of yourself and flip the thought around immediately, repeating a positive statement. For example:

I am not safe	becomes	*I have everything I need.*
I am not heard	becomes	*I am heard and acknowledged.*
I am not worthy	becomes	*I am enough.*
I am not liked	becomes	*I am lovable.*
I am not good enough	becomes	*I am magnificent.*
I am not successful	becomes	*I have achieved so much.*

Remember to use your wristband to catch and modify your inner dialogue and reactions.
So, to recap …

- ✓ Catch your reactions; can you connect your reactions to any negative beliefs?

- ✓ Can you change your mind about any negative beliefs that conflict with your goals?

- ✓ Our inner dialogue contributes to our stress levels; check in with your habitual thoughts.

- ✓ A flexible mindset allows us to reimagine what can be possible in our minds, bodies and lives.

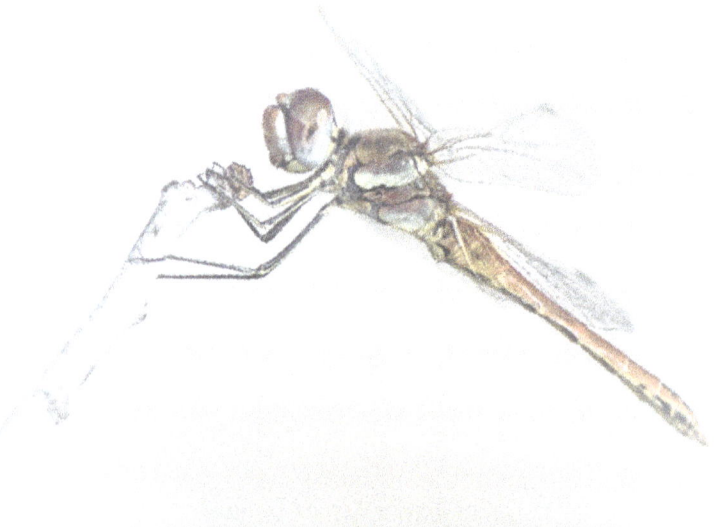

Happy body

We can strengthen the mind and body with functional restorative movement. Using active stretches and exercises, we can shift our mindset into one that promotes positivity and repair.

Happy Body is a restorative stretch and exercise program you can do at home or at work. In a kinesiology session, your physical body is assessed. A program is customised to help you manage stress and let go of any negative emotions. This session can also be delivered as an in-person or virtual presentation, or an interactive workshop for people at work, kids at school or sports athletes. More information can be found on my website.

The topics covered are:

- Nourish the mind-body connection with restorative moment
- Promote posture, fitness and detoxification
- Move the body and let go of negative emotions
- Manage stress with functional stretches and exercises

My work on movement was inspired by the body's connection to our emotional wellbeing and mental state. Using stretches and exercises, we can shift our mindset. Movement is an important daily ritual, as our muscles are connected to our brain via the nervous system.

Traditional Chinese medicine philosophy understands that our muscles are also related to our organs and emotional states. Because our mind is connected to our body, when we move our body, we are also working on our mental wellbeing. Movements allows the body to process emotions such as rage, fear and sadness. Movement can also promote positive emotions such as joy, personal power and support.

Movement helps the body to detoxify the systems of the body and organs. It promotes mobility, strength and balance in muscles, tendons, ligaments and fascia. Exercise boosts our energy and delivers oxygen and nutrients to our tissues, as well as helping our cardiovascular system to work more efficiently.

In the Happy Body program, I include vital stretching techniques and a movement program that can be done in a small space with little or no equipment. When you are stretching your body, you are also working on your mental wellbeing, personal power, your ability to let go of stress, difficult emotions and the sense of feeling stuck. Using functional stretches and exercises, we can elevate our mindset so we can process daily stress and optimise our health.

Restorative movement vs. strength and endurance

Regular exercise is one of the best tools you can use to fast track your recovery. You might be tempted to use the excuse that you are time poor; however, studies have shown that interval training in short 10-minute bursts, 2-3 times a week, can be just as beneficial as daily exercise.

To keep you motivated and make sure you're doing the most beneficial exercise for your body and lifestyle, find a strength and endurance exercise professional, such as a functional trainer, who can tailor a custom plan for you. If you are recovering from trauma or an alarmed state, you might also consider a balance of restorative exercise vs. strength and endurance. Ensure you're exercising all the different parts of your body as a whole, rather than in isolation. If you have mobility limitations, exercising in water is low impact and allows you to train muscles concentrically and eccentrically.[34]

Less is more

The good news is that, in some cases, doing less can be better because it can bring our body back to homeostasis faster. This is particularly true if you are in an alarmed state, when vigorous exercise may lead to more stress and inflammation.

In a world where we are constantly striving to push forward and achieve more, we are under so much pressure. This leads to both physical inflammation and worry because the mind and the body mirror each other. It's also important to focus on exercising your mind and your body as a whole. Achieving a 'yin' approach, by doing less and focusing on inner work, can lead to a better state of mind, better level of health, and may even assist in weight loss and a reduction in inflammation.

Movement and mindset

By exercising your body physically, you are also simultaneously working on your emotional wellbeing. This is because your muscles are connected to your brain via the nervous system, which then communicates with your organs. Each of your muscle and organ groups are

---

34 - Resistance training involves two types of movements: concentric and eccentric. Concentric movement is when the muscle shortens while producing force (contracting the muscle). This happens when you are raising the weight during a bicep curl. Eccentric movement is when the muscle lengthens while producing force.

related to emotional states, which can be identified using kinesiology.

Movement fires recovery processes in muscles and neurons. Move and stretch daily, for a stronger mind and integrated emotional health. Movement is connected to our:

- mental and emotional state
- biochemistry (hormones, cells, neurotransmitters, brain integration, gut health)
- physical body (fascia, tendons, ligaments, nerves, blood)
- qi and energy (meridians and the ability to connect to our intuition)

Many of the symptoms associated with MS can be reduced through physical exercise. Exercise is a great way to stay strong, control weight, improve fitness, and reduce the impact of specific MS symptoms.[35] The reported benefits of regular physical activity include:

- reduced fatigue levels
- improved endurance (cardiovascular fitness)
- improved balance and coordination
- improved muscle strength
- improved posture and flexibility
- improved mood, confidence and sense of wellbeing
- improved alertness and concentration
- improved ability to do everyday tasks
- reduced risk of falls
- optimised symptom recovery after a relapse
- increased energy levels

---

35 - https://www.msaustralia.org.au/news/exercise-and-ms/

While managing the symptoms of MS, exercise represents a crucial tool and is an important approach for improving health and wellness. Unfortunately, inactivity invites symptoms such as fatigue, poor strength and poor fitness. If someone is feeling fatigued, they might be less likely to exercise and as a result, they will have even more fatigue over time. Being inactive also raises the risk of developing other chronic health conditions. If you remain inactive alongside MS, you are at an increased risk of developing heart disease or diabetes too.

There is scientific evidence that exercise is associated with meaningful outcomes for people with MS, and these outcomes range from the cellular level right through to effects on quality of life. Research has indicated that people with MS who engage in exercise have better brain health based on magnetic resonance imaging (MRI), better thinking and memory (cognition), and increased mobility and cardiovascular health. Plus, people with MS who engage in exercise have less fatigue, depression, anxiety, pain, better sleep quality and quality of life.

Here are some examples of how the Happy Body movement program targets emotional wellbeing with movement.

Lunge stretch

This stretch targets the psoas muscle (hip flexor) and is great for releasing fear and a lack of motivation. It can help us to feel supported emotionally and physically, boosting our ability to move forward.

1. In a lunge position with your front foot in line with your knee.
2. Tuck your tail under and flatten your lower back curve. Slowly move your bodyweight forward keeping the body squared to the front.
3. Reach up with one arm opposite to your kneeling side and lengthen up the body.

4. To maximise the stretch tilt your body to your leading leg and rotate towards it.

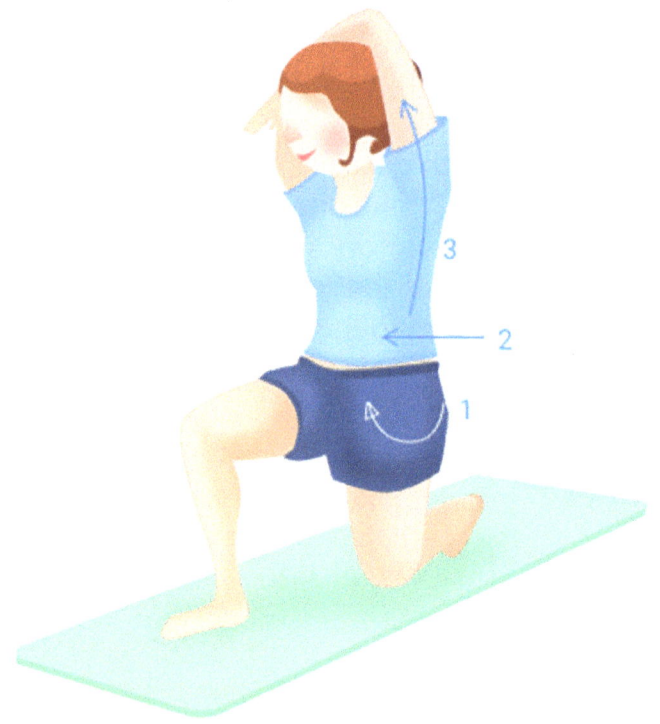

Squatting

This is a great exercise for strengthening the hips and glutes. This movement can boost self-support and the ability to receive more support in our lives. While you are squatting, think about feeling deeply supported within yourself, receiving support from your environment and your relationships. The mind and the body are connected, working on your hips which structurally support you, can boost the feeling of support within yourself, strengthening your belief that it is so.

What we believe is what matters. When we begin to believe we can support ourselves, and that we are also supported by others, we can receive more support in your life. This can enable us to see our life with fresh eyes. Our brain can seek more evidence in our environment to align with what we are focused on.

Focus on **feeling supported** and you will see more evidence of this around you. When you can believe in yourself, others will believe in you too. Keep moving, then watch possibilities open for you in your mind, body and life.

Emotional benefits

In the Happy Body online program, I've included a mind-body stretch and movement workout that helps you to destress and process your emotions all at the same time. The very special and unique part of my movement program is the emotional work you will be doing while you are working out. Each exercise and stretch targets specific muscles, and I have included the emotions that are related to those muscles.

To explore more on how to promote a happy body, you can find more information in the Appendix at the back of the book.

So, to recap ...

- ✓ Restorative movement is great for days when you are stressed.

- ✓ Stretching and exercising can help us manage stress and let go of negative emotions.

- ✓ Movement helps to promote posture, fitness and detoxification.

- ✓ Regular interval training, less can be more, promoting weight loss and a healthy cardiovascular system.

Happy food

When we eat better, we feel better. When we nourish our bodies on a cellular level, we maximise repair, transforming our mind, body and life.

Happy Food is a session that can help you to understand what foods to focus on increasing, and which ones you may want to eliminate. Healthy and delicious recipes are shared with you, including research from leading worldwide specialists. In a kinesiology session, we discover what nutrients you may need to increase to optimise repair. This session can also be delivered as an in-person or virtual presentation, or an interactive workshop for people at work, kids at school or sports athletes. More information can be found on my website.

The topics covered are:

- Nourish the body on a cellular level for repair and performance
- What foods to increase to feel good and promote repair
- Master 625 recipes
- When you eat better, you feel better

I believe that every meal can be an opportunity to renew ourselves. Nutrition is the foundation for the health of our brain, hormones and gut health, as well as our emotional and physical wellbeing.

Our body depends on water and nutrients to survive. Hydration is so important. Every cell, tissue and organ needs water to function optimally. Water makes up 90% of our lungs, 76% of our brain, 25% of our bones, 75% of our muscles that move our body, and 82% of our blood that transports nutrients.[36] Our body uses water to maintain its temperature, remove waste and lubricate joints. Our brain, muscles, skin and organs are all made up of water.

Just to perform our daily tasks, we require water and nutrients to think, walk, run and problem-solve. I recommend drinking x 8 glasses (2 litres) of water a day and make it fun. Add lemon to your water for flavour, which also promotes digestion. I love to stock my home and office with beautiful teas, so I am sipping on them all day long.

When should I increase my nutrients?

If you are going through change and a difficult time emotionally, if stress levels are high, if you have a disease and your body needs repair, I highly recommend ramping up your nutrient intake.

When I started to increase my nutrient intake, I had profound results. I've had to tweak my nutrition at different stages of my recovery. For example, I had to repair my gut before I could tolerate the various types of foods needed to maximise my nutrients. Nailing your nutrients can be a very individual and personalised process.

My goal for this chapter is to share generalised advice as well as the common denominators I have learnt over the years from various studies, doctors, research and personal experience.

To customise a specific approach that is right for you, I recommend working with a nutritionist and a naturopath, who can support your specific needs. There are biochemical tests that these practitioners can do, helping you to work out what foods are best for where your body and health journey is at.

36   Dr Libby Weaver, Internationally Acclaimed Nutritional Biochemist, Author & Speaker ~ https://www.drlibby.com

Having said that, there are fun ways to eat better. And when you eat better, you feel better, which will help you to adjust along the journey. A happy mind is connected to a happy body, when we are nourishing it with **happy foods**.

I have learned many tricks that can help you along the way, and that's what I'd love to share with you. To maximise repair in my brain, my journey led me to research and discover doctors who had their own personal stories of success and recovery. Their resources can be found on my website. I also have ebooks with delicious recipes, all designed to nourish your body on a cellular level.

It was an absolute game changer when I optimised my nutrition. Within a few months, my health and overall feeling in my mind and body had vastly improved. I no longer had to lie down for half the day, which was life-changing. I had more energy to walk and jog every few days. My MS symptoms started to completely subside. Emotionally, I started to get the spring back in my stride, the sparkle back in my eye. For me, this was proof that when you eat better you feel better, and perhaps because of my disease, this was even more noticeable. I began to fall in love with cooking and nourishing my body, a habit and attitude that translated into other areas of my life.

I came across the science behind nutrient-dense foods from the research and personal experience of doctors, and was particularly inspired by the ones who had been through their own journey of recovery from disease or trauma. With medical backgrounds, they have managed to properly research their results, and some have also conducted clinical trials. I particularly combined the work of Prof. George Jelinek[37], Dr. Terry Wahls[38], Dr. Roy Swank[39], Dr.

---

37 - https://overcomingms.org/about-us/professor-george-jelinek

38 - https://terrywahls.com/

39 - http://www.swankmsdiet.org/

John McDougal[40] and Dr. Robynne Chutkan.[41] Their work has helped many people from all over the world.

These doctors from around the globe have conducted studies on foods that successfully maximise repair, and foods which typically lead to inflammation. Our bodies are all unique and what works for one person may not be as effective for another. In my program I share the common denominators that these experts recommend, together with my approach for keeping things simple and achievable each day.

Common denominators

According to research, over 75% of Australians are not getting their recommended daily intake (RDI) of 5 servings of vegetables and 2 servings of fruit a day.[42] And when we are recovering from stress, adversity (emotional or physical), or from disease or pain, we need **more** than the RDI of nutrients, vitamins and minerals to support the process of recovery. Some studies show that we need up to 9 cups of fruit and vegetables a day to maximise repair!

In 2018, the Australian Health report found more than 99% of children and 96% of adults don't eat the RDI of 5 servings of vegetables a day.[43] And as we now know, when we need repair, we need more than the RDI of nutrients.

---

40 - https://www.drmcdougall.com/

41 - https://robynnechutkan.com/

42 - https://www.aihw.gov.au/reports/australias-health/australias-health-2018/contents/indicators-of-australias-health/fruit-and-vegetable-intake

43 - https://www.aihw.gov.au/reports/australias-health/australias-health-2018-in-brief/contents/what-can-we-improve

In my Happy Food online program, I run through a summary of the common denominators of what foods to eat and avoid, so you can ensure that you are nourishing yourself on a cellular level, maximising repair.

Where our food comes from matters

To maximise nutrients, source organic, ethical, free-range foods. Going organic helps to minimise pesticides, toxins and added hormones in our food. Ethically sourced real wholefoods are richer in antioxidants, vitamins, minerals and fibre. Think sustainable, free-range, fresh and local. Wholefoods refer to food in its most natural state.

Remember that when we drink coffee, it sends a signal to our adrenal glands to release adrenaline, which can exacerbate stress feeling more wired or 'on' in our nervous system. Particularly on days when you are more stressed, try and limit yourself to one coffee a day or remove it from your routine altogether, until you feel more balanced within.

Master 625 recipes

Master 5 salads x 5 sides x 5 sauces x 5 proteins and put all these favourite recipes in a folder. Then when you mix and match them, you have **625 recipes**! Matt Kennedy, an amazing chef, taught me that. It is how we created our menu, when I co-founded a food delivery business called *Nourissh* in 2014.

Make it fun, focus on what to increase, then organise yourself to make cooking work for you. Remember that when you eat better, you will feel better. When you feel better, you are more inclined to make better choices, leading to a happier and healthier you.

I have loads of delicious recipes in my *Happy Food eBook* that you get with the Happy Food online program, all which can be found on my website. Mindfully crafted with chefs Matt Kennedy and David Selex, these recipes are all designed to nourish our body on a cellular level. You can swap any of the proteins out with one that you prefer, or you can transform any of the dishes into a pescatarian/vegetarian/vegan dish.

To explore more on how to nourish your body with nutrition, you'll find more information in the Appendix at the back of the book.

So, to recap …

- ✓ Nourish your body on a cellular level with a variety of whole foods, greens, colour, good fats and hydration.

- ✓ Master 625 recipes with x 5 salads x 5 sides x 5 sauces x 5 proteins, mix and match.

- ✓ Reduce sugar, alcohol, coffee, red meat, processed foods and identify food allergies.

- ✓ Eat organic – where our food comes from matters.

Connection

When we are connected, we give ourselves the best environment to adapt to change and repair. Mindset tools can help you to switch off the fight or flight response, so that you can feel more positive and creative.

Connection is a session that can help you to reconnect back to yourself and within your relationships. In a kinesiology session, you will learn mindset techniques that can help you to destress and quieten your mind. This session can also be delivered as an in-person or virtual presentation, or an interactive workshop for people at work, kids at school or sports athletes. More information can be found on my website.

The topics covered are:

- Give yourself the best environment to adapt and perform
- Wash and empty the mind
- Reconnect back to yourself and within your relationships
- The power of meditation
- Fostering creativity and innovation at work

When we nourish a happy mind with a happy body with flexibility, movement and optimal nutrition, we can promote repair and growth signals in our body. As a result, we create a deeper **connection** to our internal environment (our brain, mind, cells and systems of the body). Our external environment also benefits – in particular, our connection to those around us, including our loved ones.

When we are more connected to ourselves and those we care about, we feel happier and healthier, which further helps us promote a state of repair and homeostasis in the body. From this place, we more easily connect to others with compassion, empathy and understanding, promoting a kinder world.

The benefits of connection

When we connect, there are so many benefits:

- ✓ We are more inclined to adapt to change.
- ✓ We will be kinder to ourselves and to others.
- ✓ Our body promotes repair.
- ✓ We feel happier.
- ✓ We see obstacles as opportunities.
- ✓ We are guided to make decisions from our gut instinct.
- ✓ We are more innovative, productive and engaged at work.

From a place of inner connectedness, we can achieve a higher understanding, flying above the turbulence of life, avoiding being bogged down in the chaos of inevitable change and disruption.

While learning to look after myself had been essential for my recovery, I've also discovered that having a maintenance program and maintaining consistency has helped me when I have been in a fast paced environment with work. Whether you are on top of your game wanting to optimise your performance, are needing to repair or are going through change in your life, giving yourself the best environment to thrive can really help. Consistency is key and feeling connected means you will enjoy the journey along the way.

Meditation

In our early years, as we navigate life and its changes – the highs and the lows – we tend to seek answers and connection from external sources. However, when adversity comes, we are forced to go within. I believe that everything we seek externally must be found within ourselves first. Our setbacks can end up being gifts, allowing us to awaken, to connect to the power we have within ourselves, and to heal.

Meditation is a time when we can quieten our mind. With a quiet mind, guidance comes. A regular routine is an opportunity to go within, boosting our internal anchor. This is how we can strengthen our mind, giving ourselves the best environment to achieve a higher understanding, to see our life and any challenges from the higher perspective of a mountain top. A broader perspective allows us to understand more about our situation, so we are less reactive and more open to noticing the possibility surrounding us.

A daily practice of meditation can shift our approach to setbacks, to how we deal with change and more difficult times. Wouldn't it be lovely to see them as a wonderful detour, designed to change the course of our lives, towards a new path where we are ready to walk?

We love the familiar, and we love surety. But without the ability to be resilient, which also allows us to get out of our comfort zone, to expand, to learn and to grow, a part of us dies on the inside. The processes that we go through to overcome adversity are actually teaching us to become a whole new version of ourselves.

So, can we welcome change as a good thing, even if it feels unfamiliar? It takes practice to make the unfamiliar our new normal. An elevated state brings clarity. It is like seeing your life from the top of a mountain, allowing you to achieve a higher understanding of what is going on.

I believe we are here to experience expansion and awakening. We need challenges for us to grow and get there. Challenges can be hard, but when we know what we don't want, this births desire within us and is a catalyst for creation, inspiring us to create what we **do** want. When the soul can grow, it feels expansive, we experience joy, we forgive, we can heal, we are more open to possibility and can embrace the lessons.

I love Bruce Lipton's electrical metaphor of energy and its power to heal.[44] He explains that each cell in the body is like a battery, with a negative charge on the inside and a positive charge on the outside. We have 1.4 volts of electricity in each cell, and we have 50 trillion cells. That means we have 700 trillion volts of electricity in our body in any given moment, and we can use meditation to train that energy for healing.

There is a sense of freedom when we own and take responsibility for our lives and our reality. With awareness comes choice, and with choice we can take responsibility. With greater awareness and empowerment, we can reset and rewire the brain – we really are that powerful. We are always creating with our thoughts, words and actions.

You wash your body every day. I encourage you to take the same approach with your mind. How do you wash your mind? By removing negative thoughts, old redundant ideas and habits that are no longer serving your growth, using the power of meditation. This is what allows you to become a master at letting go. It clears the space in your mind and in your life, to receive all the things that you are asking for.

---

44 - https://www.brucelipton.com/resource/article/the-wisdom-your-cells

In the Connection session, I guide you through a meditation that you can do in the morning and evening, to wash and empty your mind. Start with 10-15 mins and extend this to 20-30 minutes over time.

Body scan meditation

Every day I use my time on my mat to ask for guidance. I ask a question and sit with it, to see what messages come to me. A body scan meditation helps you to be more present, reconnecting to your body and your higher self.

After taking time to focus on my breath, I sit still for 10-20 minutes to slow down in my mind and body. From there, I imagine my crown chakra is connecting to my higher self and soul star chakra.[45] You can imagine this connection of energy is like a bubble of light, protecting you.

Then I visualise myself sitting on top of a mountain, seeing my life from this higher perspective. I ask my higher self: *What do I need to know and understand?* You can ask anything you want, and your inner guidance will come with practice.

When we exercise our energy in meditation, we can recharge just like a battery. We can strengthen our vitality, discovering that all the answers are within.

Top Tip!

Share wisdom, not baggage.

Let go of stress and negativity.

---

[45] - The Soul Star chakra connects you with your spirit and higher self. It is known as the 'seat of the soul' because it is the point where divine love and spiritual energies enter the body. The Soul Star chakra relates to spirituality, compassion and divine wisdom. We work with this chakra when we want to connect the soul to the conscious mind, understanding our purpose and ourselves better.

Visualisation

At the end of my meditation, I like to do a visualisation. I recommend you to start your day by visualising the coming weeks and months. Can you imagine the best-case scenario? Daydream it; can you feel that situation coming to you and the joy it will bring to your heart? Then as you get up, start your day believing it is so.

Role-play like you are an actor in a movie, who has just been given a script. What would you wear, how would you walk, how would you talk, if you were role-playing this new version of yourself? This is a wonderful morning ritual I use to elevate my state and vibration, so I can rise above and become greater than my fears, worries or ailments.

Practise setting your morning up for success with this elevated mindset. With an elevated state, you can connect to your higher self, and all the guidance that it provides. Power is a common theme in all our choices. When you don't know what to do, I recommend asking your higher self, from this higher view: *Will this decision empower or disempower me? Am I maintaining my power, or am I exhausting it by making this choice?*

Think of your power as currency and spend it mindfully, with all your choices, thoughts and reactions.

To explore more on meditation and connection, you'll find more information in the Appendix at the back of the book.

So, to recap …

- ✓ Wash and empty the mind with a meditation ritual morning and night.
- ✓ Reconnect back to yourself and within your relationships.
- ✓ Connection promotes growth and repair.
- ✓ Connection promotes adaptability, compassion and performance.

Journaling and gratitude

Enjoy a morning and evening ritual of journaling; set daily intentions to focus on what you want so you can make them happen. By closing the tabs within the mind and washing your mind of old stories, we can remove redundant and limiting beliefs. Elevate your mindset with intention and gratitude.

The Journaling and Gratitude session can help you to close the tabs in your mind. In a kinesiology session, you will learn a journaling technique that can help you to let go of stress and overthinking. Journaling can help us to promote gratitude, helping us to be accountable for our wellbeing. This session can also be delivered as an in-person or virtual presentation, or an interactive workshop for people at work, kids at school or sports athletes. More information can be found on my website.
The topics covered are:

- Rewire the mind to be positive and solution-focused
- Close the tabs in your mind regularly
- Reduce stress and become aware of your blind spots

Like meditation, journaling is a tool to help us wash and empty our minds and let go of stress and bad habits, like overthinking, that only lead to suffering and confusion. Journaling is a simple but effective tool that can amplify your results. It allows you to measure your progress and keeps you on track. I love journaling and use this ritual every morning and night, to set up my focus and adjust my state.

In my Journaling online session, I have a journal with morning and evening questions that help you to identify what your barriers are, so you can work through them on paper. This helps you to be more aware of what to focus on, which sets up your brain to notice more opportunities around you.

Rewiring the brain

What we think and believe are a mirror image of our reality and the health of our bodies. We can leverage the power of our brain to heal and make things happen for ourselves.

The brain is an amazing control centre. It oversees our conscious and subconscious processes, allowing us to navigate life. Earlier in the book, we explored the reticular activating system (RAS). We can work with this amazing filter system to rewire our brain. The brain processes approximately 400 billion bits of information a second, and only 2,000 of those consciously, so we need a filter system.

Let's look at some examples of the RAS at work. You may have a new car on your mind – let's pretend it's a white Lexus. Now that a white Lexus is in your focus, you may notice more of them on the road than before. That is because your RAS is doing its job! Another example is when a new mum notices more baby ads on TV or overhears more conversations about babies. The ads and conversations have always been there; however, we do notice more of what we are focused on in our environment.

The RAS can be leveraged to focus on what we want, opening our perceptions to see more opportunities around us. The same is true for negative emotions: when anger, fear or self-doubt are in our focus, we find more evidence of this around us. This also becomes the lens that we see our world through.

Using journaling, we can make a conscious effort to focus on what we want, getting really clear on what that is for us. This clarity and focus can be very healing and productive. Daily journaling can help you notice more opportunities to bring what you want into your life.

Take a moment now to reflect on what you value and what you would like to bring into your life, regarding love, health, family, career and finances. Are you clear on what you want in the next year, in 5 years, in 10 years?

Making a vision board can be a great way to discover what you want, setting up your brain to notice opportunities around you. Your environment and private spaces are also your 3D vision boards. Clear your spaces regularly and surround yourself with whatever evokes joy for you.

You have all the power within you; all the solutions that you have looked for externally exist within you. You already have all the answers. As you begin to see your life with fresh eyes and through a new lens, you may notice your reactions change. You are calmer, you may feel more connected within you.

Welcome to the power of journaling. I know that it can be a pivotal addition to help you overcome anything you are going through. Remember, consistency will elevate your energy, so you can see your life from that higher perspective, from the top of a mountain, with a higher understanding of your mind, hurdles and life. This is the best environment you can give yourself to repair and thrive.

To explore more on journaling and the morning and evening questions that I ask myself, you'll find more information in the Appendix at the back of the book.

The Bend Like Bamboo program can give you all the tools you need to take action. When we become aware of any suppressed inner conflict, it becomes empowering.

From there we can understand why we are where we are, and how we got there. With this awareness, we can move forwards and take responsibility to transform our mind, body and life.

So, to recap …

- ✓ Journaling reduces stress and helps us to process the day.

- ✓ Close the tabs in your mind with a daily journaling ritual.

- ✓ Create a life with gratitude and intention.

- ✓ Journaling helps us be accountable and review positive and negative habits.

Bend Like Bamboo for work, school and sports performance

Sometimes the workplace needs a reset. To overcome change, stress and disconnection. To take the time to reconnect and realign. I believe that flexibility builds resilience and, in turn, building resilience in people improves business. I work with CEOs, leaders, kids and athletes to help them master resilience, uncover blind spots, and achieve their personal and professional goals.

A flexible attitude impacts on everything that comes our way. Being open to change can have an enormous positive impact on the work environment, leading to improved relationships and quality project outcomes.

Business productivity and performance are lifted when teams become more resilient and quickly identify stress and negative patterns. Understanding and mastering this benefits employees and employers alike.

The *Bend Like Bamboo* resilience program is available in-person and online, and can be customised for workplaces and schools, as well as athletes, around Australia and globally.

From my experience

After launching two businesses in the short space of two years, as the CEO I had to be on top of my game to perform at my best. I found that the same techniques I used to rebuild my life, when recovering from paralysis, also applied to optimising my business performance. This helped me to maintain a fast-paced environment at a time when I had to be creative and innovative, in the start-up phase of the businesses.

I am passionate about resilience and happiness at work, because I know how burnout can feel. We can perform in a more balanced way that leads to better productivity, engagement and innovation. When we are happy at work, we feel healthier and more resilient.

A growth mindset is a state that becomes contagious, especially within a work culture. We are all so connected; when one person or team drops communication and becomes stressed, it impacts on the whole structure. Looking after ourselves personally translates into our professional lives; when we feel like a leader, we think and act like a leader too.

We all want to experience fulfilment in our personal lives. At work, where we spend 50% or more of our time, we want to stretch ourselves professionally, so that we can perform at our best and reach our full potential.

How Bend Like Bamboo can help you

Ask yourself the following questions:

- Are you feeling stressed, unmotivated, exhausted or unwell?
- Are you lacking in self-belief and self-confidence?
- Are you attracting loving and supportive relationships?
- Is your life unfolding in a way that aligns with what you really want?
- Is fear your default reaction; do you focus on the risks and the negatives?
- Do you get stuck in your head, overthinking and overanalysing?
- Are you sabotaging your success, unable to make things happen for you?
- Does every morning feel like Groundhog Day; are you living on autopilot?
- Or do you simply want to make a particular change in your life?

Having a goal is not enough to make it happen. **What we believe is what matters**. We can feel stress, or we could be experiencing change from experiences e.g., a lack of money, feeling powerless, out of control, going through a divorce, a break-up or a change in job. Sometimes change is exciting and manageable, but sometimes it can totally blow our circuits.

When we are stressed, we focus more on the negative, we can over-worry, we are more rigid, unhappy and unwell. We squeeze out the fun and joy from what we are doing, we overthink and get stuck in our heads. We are disengaged, unkind and cannot perform at our best.

When we are having more fun and believing in ourselves, we can make things happen. We are more flexible, we are solution-focused, we are more connected. Our energy is more elevated, and this is powerful.

When we have a goal, but our beliefs are not in alignment, it feels like a push/pull; you know how it feels when you really want something but are too scared to go for it, or are not believing in yourself. An inner resistance builds and builds and becomes background stress that lingers. When you feel like this, it is a time to ask yourself: *Do I believe in myself? Do I believe I can make it happen? And do I believe that I deserve it?* If not, can you change your mind about this 'story'?

This 'inner conflict' is also a cause of stress. I learned this on my own journey and in my private practice seeing clients with body pain, digestive issues, anxiety, depression and various diseases. A stress caused by inner conflict sends a stress response from our brain out to our biochemistry to freeze, flight or fight.

If how we think and feel is connected to the biochemistry of our bodies and the stress response, is there a way to promote repair and growth pathways instead that can help us to destress, allowing us to feel more creative, solution-focused, adaptable and flexible?[46]

Discovering your inner conflict can be a game changer for you. It can unleash you from sabotage, poor health and

---

46 - Bruce H. Lipton, Ph.D., cell biologist and lecturer, is an internationally recognised leader in bridging science and spirit. He is the bestselling author of *The Biology of Belief* and *The Honeymoon Effect*.

unhappiness. As the practitioner and the patient, I have learned that our inner conflicts are often left unaddressed, as we are not always aware of them. That is because what we believe is a very subconscious process.

It is not just the consumption of unhealthy food and a lack of exercise that can cause stress. It is also how we are feeling about ourselves, our belief in ourselves, and our ability to make things happen in our lives. I highly recommend finding a practitioner who works with the subconscious brain, as in kinesiology, to help you to discover any inner conflict within you.

The inner conflict

We all have experienced an inner conflict, when what we believe is not aligning with what we want. It could be from fear of starting a new business, receiving more love in our life, or moving on from a situation that is no longer right for us.

When we ignore inner conflict, it can brew up inside us; it can make us tired, as we spend a lot of energy battling the resistance. Instead of fighting what we are resisting, can we use the resistance and this inner frustration as a catalyst that can propel us forward to grow and become more?

Have you ever felt that inner conflict within you? When you know what you need to do, you may even know what action you should take, but there is a part of you that holds back. You might fear that things won't work out, that you won't handle the change. You might make excuses and find ways to legitimately believe them. When we feel afraid, we can forget the truth and what we are capable of and lose access to the resources we have within. They can be accessed the second we choose to step up and face our fears. We often don't find these hidden gems within us until we are forced to go within, from adversity, tragedy or forced change.

When I have sat in my inner conflict, not yet ready to step up, I knew it in the depths of my being. My body also communicated with me, with a sore neck, back, anxiety or more dramatic symptoms that debilitated me, like paralysis and crushing fatigue. Here are some examples of beliefs and how they can be mirrored by our actions:

Belief	Behaviour
Belief that I am not successful	Will work overtime without an off button.
Belief that I am not lovable	You find it hard to receive love and support.
Belief I am not beautiful or sexy	You find it hard to put yourself out there, to date or meet people.
Belief that others aren't trustworthy	You block new love and friendships.
Belief that you will be let down	You have become overly self-sufficient.

Chapter 11
Ideas vs. Beliefs

An idea is a goal or a desire e.g., I want success, better health, or to bring more love into my life. Our inner conflict is when we have an idea or goal, but it conflicts with what we believe about ourselves or what can be possible for us.

Align your goals with positive beliefs

Do you take the time to go within and regularly listen to your inner voice? We can't escape it, but we sure do try. We numb ourselves with being busy, drinking alcohol or taking sedatives, addictions which sabotage behaviour and lead us to lose touch with our inner guidance.

When was the last time you questioned your beliefs? It's worth taking time on a regular basis to consciously reconcile your goals with your beliefs. It can be very powerful. As I've said throughout the book, what we believe is what matters: it determines how we react, how we perceive our environment, how stressed we are and the health of our bodies. If we don't check in and question our beliefs, we can end up living our entire life from a story that may not be true for us, simply because we have not reviewed old perceptions and let go of the past.

When I was young, I developed beliefs that I wasn't approved of; I have spent much of my life striving too much as a result. It's exhausting. Living and thinking this way led me to overwork, as it felt like a matter of life or death, how

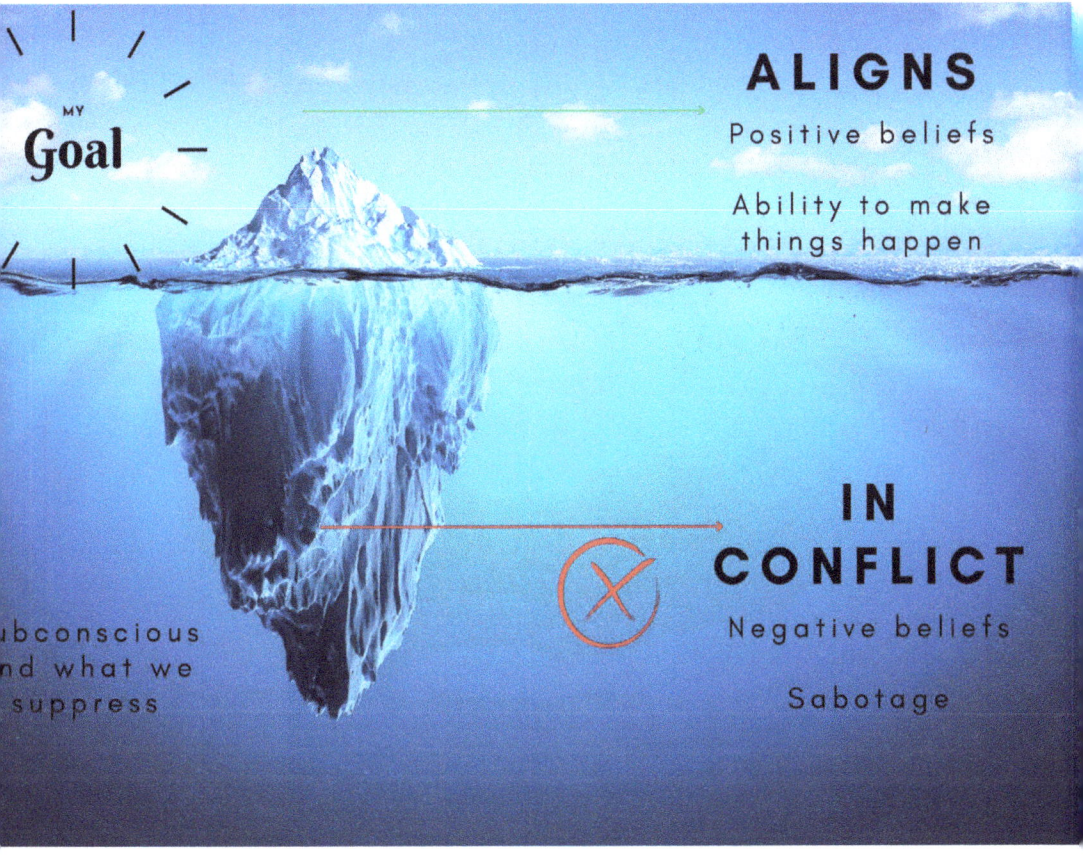

The inner conflict vs. an alignment of goals and positive beliefs

much I needed to achieve in a day. Not fun, and not always productive either when it is coming from a place of fear.

Our reactions can show us what we are believing. Catch yourself in the moment when you are reacting and ask yourself: What am I believing right now? Also ask: Is this story I am telling myself even true for me anymore? And then the most important question to ask is: Can I change my mind about this?

This is the art of Bending Like Bamboo. Reimagining what can be possible for us, rising to the challenge, accepting our call to adventure, and discovering what we are made of. This is the space where miracles happen, where our superpower is revealed, where we can let go of the world as we knew it, and step into a new reality of possibility.

Get to the bottom of what has stressed you out. Knowing if you are stuck in a stress response, and when and why it started, can be a game changer when optimising health and performance. This is my number one goal when working with clients, and when working on structural, emotional and biochemical imbalances.

Address your environment. Our cells are constantly perceiving their environment. If you perceive a threat, they will signal to genes in your body and reflect in your overall health.

My turning point

Prior to my paralysis attack, I had used all my energy being upset about what was out of my control. I was being so hard on myself to achieve, despite my MS diagnosis. How I was thinking, feeling and perceiving these difficult times in my life had led to more degeneration and an acceleration of my disease.

At one of my first rehab sessions, I remember sitting in my wheelchair attempting one of the first exercises, trying to make my fingers open and close. I had tears running down my face because it was so hard! In that moment, I knew I had a choice: I could give up or ...

To get better results, I knew I had to **change my mind**, and my approach, about what I believed was possible.

Living in rehab, I was no longer distracted. I had already reached rock bottom, my fears had been realised. I was living the nightmare, so I let go of trying to control everything. My suppressed feelings began to surface, and I could feel my nervous system surrender. I dove into the darkness and instead of resisting it, I began to walk through and into it. I could only focus on each individual moment, because hour by hour I was tackling what were some of the biggest hurdles I had ever had to face. Because what I was tackling was so big, it felt much more manageable to break it down into moment-by-moment pieces. Little did I know, this forced me to live more in the present moment.

The biggest thing I learned in rehab was realising that when we just surrender and use our energy to roll up our sleeves and step into the dark abyss of the unknown, rather than using all our energy reserves procrastinating, fearing change and resisting getting out of our comfort zone, we build inner resilience. We are equipped to deal with what comes, and ironically, it can be easier than the suffering we sometimes bring into our lives, when we avoid an inevitable path that we must walk. Can you see this unfamiliar path as the way to healing, and a new life that you are ready to step into?

There were many weeks of nothing, no improvement in my condition. There were days of sitting in my wheelchair, crying behind my (very black) sunglasses. It was a waiting game, and it was so confronting. My mind would wander into negative thoughts about how bad this could get and why this was happening to me. Then to thoughts of, 'No, I cannot continue like this anymore! I will recover, this is only temporary.' I began to see my circumstances with a new perspective, giving the situation a new meaning. I asked myself, 'What do I need to learn, to get past this setback?'

With a fresh perspective, I tried to understand how this experience was happening for me. On the days when I went into a black hole, I would only allow myself to entertain my worst fears in the company of my twin sister, and we held hands and cried. It was one of the hardest, darkest times of my life.

Chapter 12
The Pineapple Effect

In my life, I have faced situations that have tested my resilience. I have found it beneficial to catch myself when stress can lead to an overreaction. Our reactions are malleable and can be an opportunity for us to choose a new one. This is also a way we can train the brain to let go of the old story that may be old and redundant. Our reactions can also be an amazing mirror that can expose what we are really believing about ourselves and what can be possible for our future. If how we navigate change determines our success, if our reactions are born from an accumulation of past events and what we have learned from people and the environment, can we then understand the importance of stepping into our power to choose our reactions?

Our reactions are so important; they are an opportunity to look at where we are at in our lives, emotionally and spiritually. If we use them as a tool to bring in more awareness, if we are brave enough to look at what we are ignoring, I believe this can be a catalyst for real change in the mind and body. When I did this for myself, I watched my health and life transform before my eyes, much faster than I could ever have imagined.

The Pineapple Effect is a technique I created with my twin sister. It is a safe phrase we use to nourish our relationship. She is the introvert and I am the extrovert, so this is a really helpful technique that has helped us to be kinder to each other. We use it when we catch ourselves in the moment when we are overreacting. At such times, my twin sister and I use the word 'pineapple' to defrag ourselves, to help us remember to pause in the moment. It helps when we get lost in negativity, when we lose insight and kindness, when we are in conflict, and when we are looking at a situation from a perspective that is merely reactive, rather than objective.

You can use The Pineapple Effect too. Can you catch yourself when you next overreact, by asking yourself this question: What am I believing? What am I believing about myself or this situation that is causing an overreaction within me? Maybe right now in your life, you are believing that nothing is working out for you, that you are not enough, that this moment warrants an outburst of anger. Or instead, you may want to hide away from fear.

Our reactions give us a choice of who we want to be in such moments. They are very special moments where we can:

- uncover what we are believing about ourselves and our circumstances;
- question whether our reaction is just an old habit, and whether these thoughts are even true for us anymore;
- uncover what we have suppressed that has come out in a reaction, providing an opportunity to transform any anger, guilt, fear and associated emotional pain; and then
- choose a new reaction that aligns with who we want to be and how we want to feel, letting go of any inner conflict.

Remember, when we are stressed, we tend to focus on the negative and worst-case scenarios, forgetting the positive. Diaphragm breathing is another great tool to help us feel calmer and more present in the moment – our most creative state. This action communicates a calming signal to the nervous system, which is why meditation is such a good tool to help us destress.

In our relationships

How we connect in our interpersonal relationships is something we must all deal with in our lives; how we communicate is key. We must interact with people who have opposing beliefs to us and very different personalities. It is important to acknowledge that how others see the world may be very different from the way that we do, and that's okay. We are often attracted to people who are opposite to us, as opposites attract. The power of polarity allows us to learn from what we don't want or like; how we control our emotions, stress levels and reactions is key here.

In our intimate relationships, The Pineapple Effect is a great tool that allows us to catch ourselves in the moment, when we know we are merely reacting due to conflict and not showing up to be the best version of ourselves we know we can be. When we take the time to pause and catch ourselves in our reactions, we can elevate and rise above our situation, seeing it from a bird's eye perspective. Then we can have a greater understanding of what is going on and make better decisions as a result.

Within ourselves

The Pineapple Effect is also a great tool we can use on ourselves, as we all can react negatively within ourselves, not just in our interactions with others. Try to catch yourself in your next reaction; I like using a wristband as a prop to remind me to do it. I mentioned earlier that I created my own wristbands at Bend Like Bamboo that say, 'I am enough'. I catch myself and I question: Am I seeing this from fear or a negative mindset? Can I anchor back within myself, can I reconnect back into my heart, and see this with fresh eyes?

Have I gone into a negative dialogue? Or am I entertaining an old story because I am stressed?

I pause when I look at my wristband, as it helps to remind me to bring this moment into my awareness and let any old stories go. I replace any negative inner dialogue with positive words or a new narrative that aligns with what I am wanting in my life, and who I am wanting to be.

Self-esteem and communication are so important! Confidence and self-belief start in our minds, with thoughts, to feelings and our actions. We can get stuck in the monkey mind, and we have no idea that we are in our heads overthinking. We can go over and over negative narratives and old stories, believing that this is going to keep us safe. This typically happens when we become frightened, trust is broken, when we are pushed out of our comfort zone, when we go into shock, or when we are dealing with change. Overthinking is often linked to headaches, sore neck and shoulders and the inability to be flexible.

When we find ourselves focused on the past or overanalysing the future in the monkey mind, it can be helpful to use a prop that reminds us to consciously drop out of our heads and back into our hearts, where we can

How to Use the Pineapple Effect

1. Catch yourself in the moment with the word 'pineapple'.
2. Question your reaction and the associated thoughts/story/emotions.
3. Ask yourself: Is this an old habit? Is it really true for me anymore?
4. Choose a new reaction that aligns with what you want in your life, and the positive emotions you want to feel. When you feel good, you will be more resilient, flexible and open to change.

be calmer. From the heart space, we can be more open and loving, towards ourselves and others. We can be more compassionate, more creative, adaptable and resilient.

When we are stressed, we tend to focus on the negative and we can react by playing small, being overly cautious to feel safe. But we do not grow when we react like this. The Pineapple Effect is a tool that can help us to rewire the brain to focus on the positive. This translates to the decisions we make and how we show up in the world.

We can choose who we want to be in every moment. With awareness comes choice, and with choice comes the realisation that we are fully in charge of our mind, body and life. You can start with your reactions today. I hope you enjoy using The Pineapple Effect as much as I do.

Here are two more tips for resetting old habits:

1. Start with the smaller changes, as they will translate to the bigger ones in your life. Brush your teeth with a different hand, walk home on new routes. We can train our brain to welcome change.

2. Do something that scares you every day. This could be as simple as trying something new or choosing the option you would usually say 'no way' to. Not only will this technique give you proof that good things can happen when you get out of your comfort zone, it also amplifies neuroplasticity. I am a huge believer that whatever scares us can often be the very thing that we need to do to overcome our inner conflict.

Practising being more aware of our reactions can help us to understand what is behind them. With a more positive mindset, we can discover just how powerful we are. Every word, every thought and every choice is either empowering or disempowering you.

You can change your mind

To change our life, we must first believe it is possible. We must be able to close our eyes and see a vision of this reality, feeling and connecting to the emotions of having it and the joy it would bring into our life. It is an act of creation, forming more energy around a thought, a desire and an imagined reality, then drawing it into our life physically. What starts as an idea and the birth of a desire – usually from realising what we don't want – slowly becomes an organism that we nourish, water and grow.

After researching stories of recovery and observing results I have had, both with my clients and on my own journey, I have observed that a transformation is more likely to occur when the idea and desire for a result (conscious) shifts to a deeper (subconscious) belief that it is possible. This takes courage, vulnerability and is often a journey of learning new thoughts, habits and routines.

Just wanting something for ourselves is not enough to make it happen. I am going to repeat this again and again: what we believe is what matters. If we have lost belief in ourselves, we can change our minds about what we are believing. It is the most important thing we can do to optimise our wellbeing, so that we can build the resilience to stretch ourselves more and become what we are ready for next in our lives. If you have not yet manifested your goals yet, ask yourself have I become this within myself yet?

I believe every possible scenario has its own signature vibration. If we want to create something, we need to embody its vision like it has already happened, aligning with its energy, and therefore drawing it into our reality.

I am astounded by the power of joy. When stressed, we can block pleasure and joy from our lives, perhaps from a punishment or sabotage cycle we are familiar with or addicted to, or from something we are unaware of. Life isn't easy. We form our identity and beliefs at such a suggestible age, when our brain is still learning who we are and what we believe. Often, the pain or trauma that our ailments and issues stem from happened during our childhood. The lessons we learn along the way make us who we are, and our ability to be flexible can help us to see this with love and compassion, inspiring us to keep moving forward so that we can discover what we are made of.

Elevate your state

My wristband that I use as a prop helps me remember to get out of my head and drop into my heart, bringing myself back into the present moment to reconnect.

My hope is that you enjoy living in an anchored state, just like a bamboo tree. Feeling anchored within yourself you can notice a more flexible mindset, seeing your world from a higher perspective, with fresh eyes and a higher understanding of your life and circumstances. I believe that our setbacks, circumstances and the hurdles we face are in our lives to help us grow. I'd love for you to see each challenge as a gift, leading you to a path that will help you become the person you are ready to be, to receive all that you are wanting.

Once you master anchoring within daily, I then want you to practise capturing this state throughout the day. You should notice you are less reactive and more observant. Every word, every thought, every choice you make is creating your health and your reality. I believe you can change your mind about what can be possible for you, reimagining your health and your life.

Forgiveness

Forgiveness is an exercise of surrender that can help us to shift resistance and whatever is disconnecting us. Is there a person or an event that you think you can forgive? Is there an unresolved conflict that is taxing your energy? Any inner conflict can eat away at us; when left unresolved, the build-up of energy and pressure can manifest into symptoms such as pain, digestive issues, anxiety or even depression.

The art of forgiveness can elevate our energy, allowing more joy, love and light into our lives. Holding onto anger or grief only hurts us. We are all connected, so when we forgive someone who we perceive has hurt us, energetically we also create and hold a space for that person to be open to love and forgiveness too. You may notice the vibe shift between you and this person.

Memories from the past serve us so that we can learn from past mistakes. But when we anchor into the pain of on old story, we can overthink or identify with it, and this can affect our health. This is what I call hell on earth; we can remain stuck in a mental prison, reliving old pain over and over, and creating a reality that mirrors it. As a result, our future thoughts, perceptions and actions can lead to us reliving the past. This limiting approach prevents us from creating a new future, mind, body or life.

We limit ourselves when we anchor into shame, guilt, anger, fear, worry or envy. Can you use the power of flexibility, to let go of your story? Let it go. Can you see your situation from multiple perspectives, from a more elevated perspective? Can you then give the past a new meaning? What you may also find is that you can begin to perceive things differently, freeing you from jail. Welcome to heaven on earth, where the light turns on and you can see again. It has all been an illusion, you have been living in the dark.

I believe that everyone is doing their best at the level of consciousness that they are at on their journey. I recommend using journaling if you find it hard to forgive. This exercise can help you to get it out of your head, and onto paper. Write down what has hurt you, and what you have learned while overcoming the conflict you have faced. When you choose to forgive, you can take back your power and transform your pain.

Follow your joy

In hospital the days were long, broken only by three physio sessions a day, five days a week, and visits from my beautiful friends and family. I spent hours alone with my thoughts, unable to contemplate living life in a broken shell.

In my rehab sessions, I was surrounded by people suffering the ramifications of drug overdoses, car accidents and strokes. So much suffering, so many stories. Inspired by their stories, I was forced to re-evaluate my life and how I measured success and happiness.

I started to surrender to the flow of what each day entailed. I felt like I had a strength within me, that had always been there but had been activated, as though coming from another source. It was a sense of calm and a deep knowing, like I had never felt before. This was the first time I experienced feeling guided, as if held by an external force. It was a pivotal time in my life, and I do believe something bigger was at play here. I began to listen; I was learning who the next version of myself would be, after going through so much. But there were many weeks of no hope, no movement, no change.

When I was not exercising in rehab, or asleep from the exhaustion, I spent much of my time sitting in my wheelchair, contemplating my life and my fate. At the time I was on Avonex, a drug that you had to inject into your leg once a week (with a long intramuscular needle about an inch deep). With only one functioning hand and arm, it was difficult to inject myself. My twin sister Nicole would help me, and I worked out that if I could stretch the skin on one of my thighs with my working hand, she could hold the needle above, and on the count of three would dart it in. One day, a nurse walked in on us when we were counting down 3, 2, 1 … She looked startled, then realised what we were trying to accomplish together. She smiled with kind compassionate eyes, quietly closed the door, and let us get on with the job.

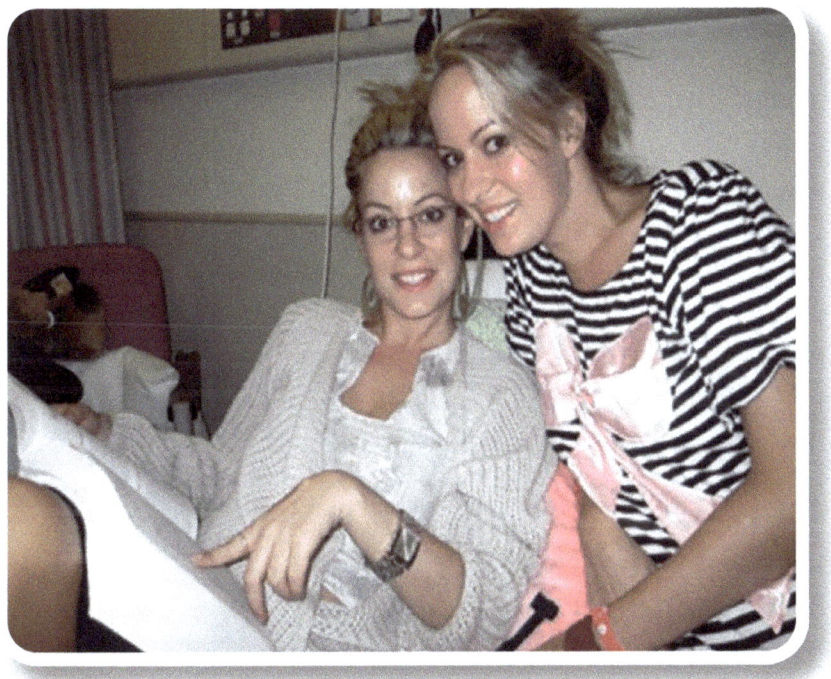

Nicole visiting and Amanda at Epworth Richmond

I found hope

Every Tuesday night, my friends and I used to have a girls' night out, which I couldn't attend while living in rehab. However, sometimes my beautiful girlfriends would come to me, and those nights were the highlight of my week – my month! It was so wonderful for me to still feel connected to my mates, while going through such an isolating, terrifying time in my life. I cannot begin to express how grateful I am to each of my mates who visited me.

I am lucky to have amazing friends. They were busy with their careers and full schedules, but they took the time to come and see me after work every few weeks. Like a scene in *The Hangover*, walking down the corridor, finishing their day talking on their mobile phones, fabulous as ever, my friends turned heads. Every time we were together, it was like an *Entourage* episode; we all had so much fun together, usually belly laughing out loud, as I was carted around the hospital in my wheelchair. I was a lucky girl and it really reminded me about the power of friendship and connection and their role when we're healing.

It goes without saying that my family were also dedicated to ensuring I had what I needed and didn't feel alone. Mum visited as often as she could, as she was at home looking after our grandmother who had been diagnosed with Alzheimer's disease not long before. Nicole would lie in my single hospital bed some nights, so I wasn't alone. In the morning, if we had a nice nurse, she would draw the curtains and say, 'Morning twins!' and bring in breakfast for two. I cannot begin to express how grateful I am for Nicole's love and kindness through this challenging time of my life.

One Tuesday night, I had dinner with some girlfriends, Teisha, Vicky, Penny, Sarah, Caz, Jane and my sister Nicole. They wheeled me out of hospital and across the road to the pub. We laughed over dinner, and I forgot about the 24/7 nightmare that was my reality. That night, I felt more joy and elation in my body than I ever had before. It was like I received and absorbed pleasure for the first time in my life. Perhaps it was because it had been so long since I'd felt happy? It was the most fun I'd had in months. I felt connected, less stressed and more present in the moment.

What I also know is that in that moment I redefined what happiness meant to me; gratitude swept up inside me and I felt it intensely in a transformative way.

It is the little things that matter most and that you miss when you lose so much in your life. Like being able to dress yourself, drive to where you need to go, and to just laugh and have cherished moments with the ones you love.

After that Tuesday night dinner, something very special happened. Nicole wheeled me back to my room and helped me change into my pyjamas. Then she went to the bathroom and suddenly, my toe on my paralysed foot moved for the first time.

In that moment, **I found hope and started to channel my energy differently**. A new motivation came over me, and I knew what I had to do! With hope, I now had the courage to focus on what I wanted, instead of what I didn't want. This shifted what I believed could be possible, and I began to use my energy towards recovery, instead of being so frightened. This was a massive transformation for me and would later translate into every other part of my life.

The next day I was first in at physio and last to leave; I was a woman on a mission. I was focused, determined and wanted to get my mind, my body and my life back. After that moment of change I felt guided, like I knew what I had to do. I had clarity and could see a path forward. Everything started to flow with momentum. I noticed my body responding more and more to physio, and I began to move other parts of my paralysed left side. The way my body was mirroring my mindset shift inspired me; it was so life-changing. This incredible gift was literally about to change every other aspect of my life. I had been given a second chance.

My suffering was reducing; I had more energy, brain integration and problem-solving capacity to navigate myself towards solutions. Feeling safer in my body, my brain let go of stress more and more. Little did I know, perhaps my brain began to prioritise growth and repair pathways, rather than survival and degeneration? The clouds began to lift – it was like an outer body experience. A strength and focus grew within me like I had never experienced before. I discovered a sense of self-belief and awakening; for the first time, I truly began to believe in myself and what I could be capable of.

A new version of myself was born, and a bright light emanated from within. Feeling safe and motivated, I had more energy to rejuvenate and heal. My perspective shifted about my circumstances, leading to a higher understanding, inviting new solutions and a renewed sense of wellbeing.

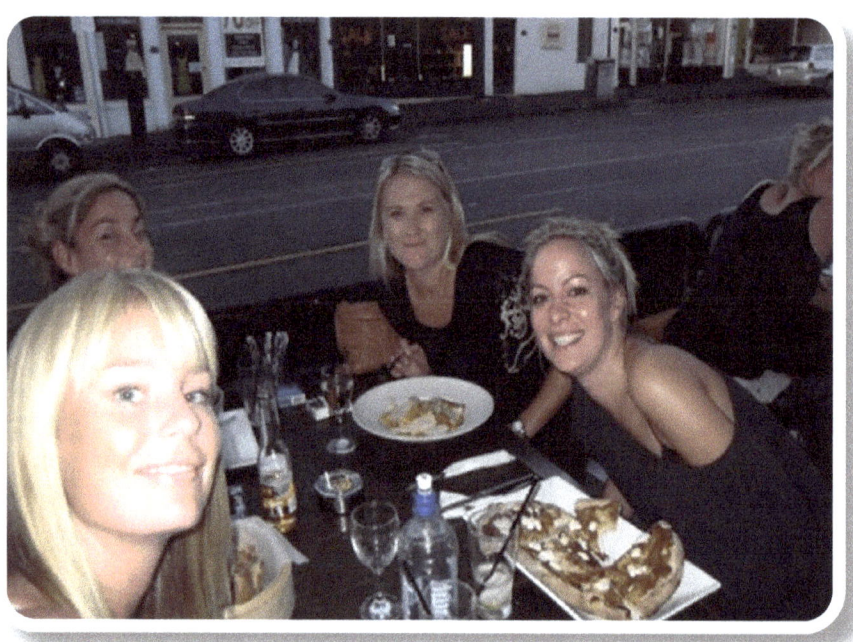

Teisha, Jane, Caz and Nicole out to dinner with me opposite the hospital the night my toe moved

I found joy

I learned about the importance of joy and the impact it can have on our mind and body. I also learned that you can only truly cherish the light of joy when you know the despair of darkness. We all go through setbacks in our lives, some easier than others, some that will completely rock you. I believe those rock-bottom moments, when we have no choice but to succeed, can serve as a catalyst for change. Perhaps those moments of contrast are part of life's design, teaching us to develop understanding and wisdom, using the power of polarity for a deeper understanding of life? I have also learned that setbacks can be detours that are designed to move us on. Maybe we are supposed to feel uncomfortable, so that we are forced to walk a new path?

As a doer and a girl who thrives when she feels driven, I did what I knew: I worked hard in my physio sessions, three times a day, five days a week. I had to relearn how to use my left hand, arm and leg again, and how to eat with two hands. I had to relearn how to wash and dry myself. I discovered that fine motor skills are quite important and necessary for lifting your hands over your head, allowing you to wash your hair. I had to relearn how to pick things up, how to smile, how to problem-solve, how to exist again. Week by week, I started to get movement back in my toes, fingers, arms, legs and face. I learned how to use a foot brace to walk, holding onto people or a wall. The leg brace helped me to lift my leg up when I began to relearn how to walk; my gait was still returning, stage by stage.

I progressed to walking with my left knee taped up, then to walking on my own! Those first few steps to freedom were … indescribable. I was walking again! There was my life before that moment, and my life after. A switch turned on inside me, and I channelled my rock-bottom moment into pure drive, and fought to get to the other side. I was determined to leave that hospital, not just walking but running!

And I did. It wasn't the most graceful of runs, but I did it.

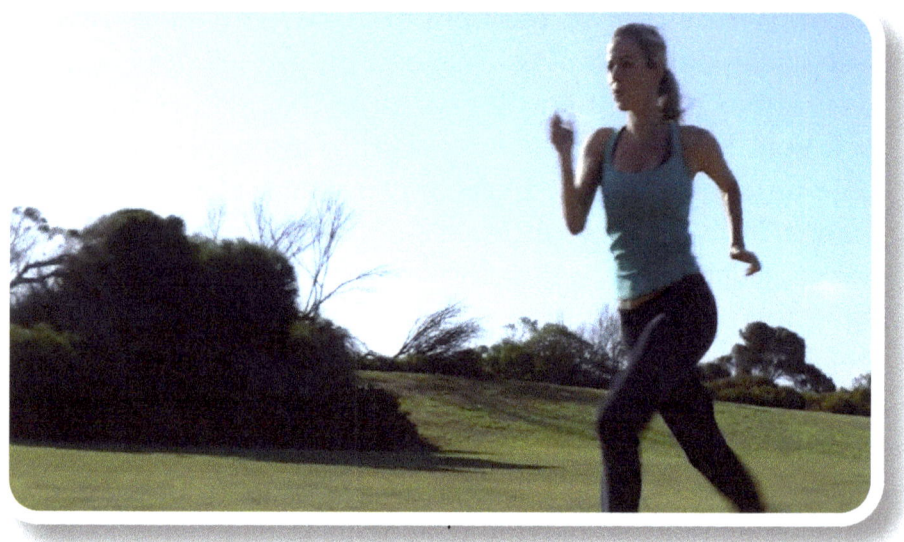

Amanda running

I went from walking to running within six weeks of the prognosis I had been given. I remember sitting with the head of neurology when I was admitted into rehabilitation, and he predicted that I may be permanently paralysed for the rest of my life. Turning my destiny around created a profound shift within me. It was the first time I fully understood what I was capable of. It was the evidence my brain needed to change my mind about what could be possible for my future and the course of my disease. This would later translate into other areas of my life, transforming how I showed up in my life.

My transformation wasn't just about me, far from it. I had an amazing team of people who helped me, and who helped me believe that I could do it. They stood with me when I couldn't stand and helped me get to where I am today. I had physios, speech therapists, counsellors, occupational therapists, neurologists, a kinesiologist, family and friends. I could not have come through this ordeal with the courage and determination that I had, if it had not been for my loving supportive family and friends – in particular, my twin sister, Nicole. She dropped everything to be there for me day and night. I count my lucky stars for her love and compassion during the hardest time of my life.

My Mum has since left this planet on Mother's Day, 9 May 2021, and I dedicate this book to her. My Mum always loved me and never judged me. No matter what, I always felt so loved by you Ma, and you inspire me to push myself to keep going, to become my fullest potential and make you proud of who I am and what I am yet to become. Because you loved me, I know real unconditional love. I still feel your love, even though you are not physically here.

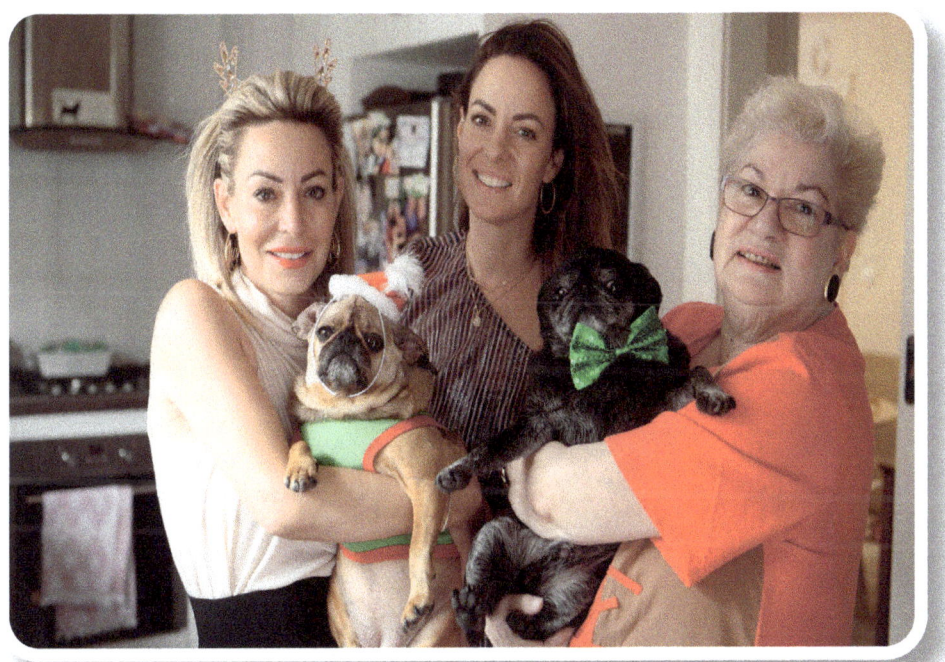

Mums and Henry's last Christmas

While I was living in hospital, all this love and support really accelerated my healing. A massive thank you to all my friends for being there with me through some of the most difficult times. It touched my heart and gave me the will to keep going.

I will forever be indebted to the exceptional neuro-physiotherapists at Epworth Richmond, Gavin and Shaun. Neuro-physiotherapy, in combination with an Eastern approach to kinesiology, would be the start of my understanding of the power of a balanced approach. The combination of Western and Eastern medicine was so effective on my journey.

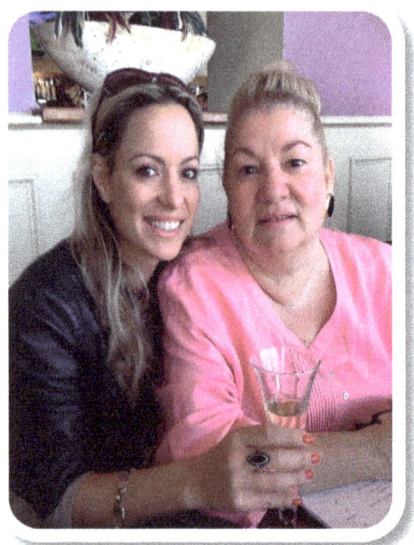

Mum and I celebrating my Kinesiology graduation at Malvern pub

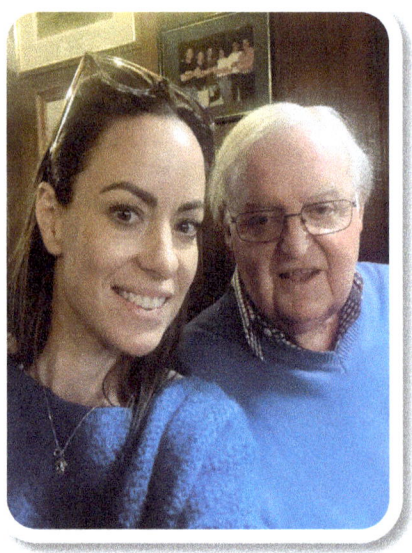

Amanda & Noel (Dad) at Romeos Toorak

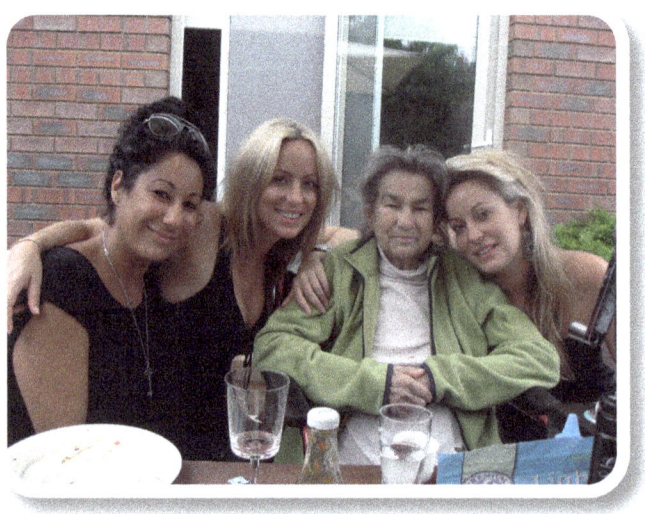

Anthea, Amanda, Grandma, and Nicole

It was amazing, experiencing my body mirroring my new outlook on life! I had no idea that this shift in my mindset was altering my biochemistry. It was instrumental

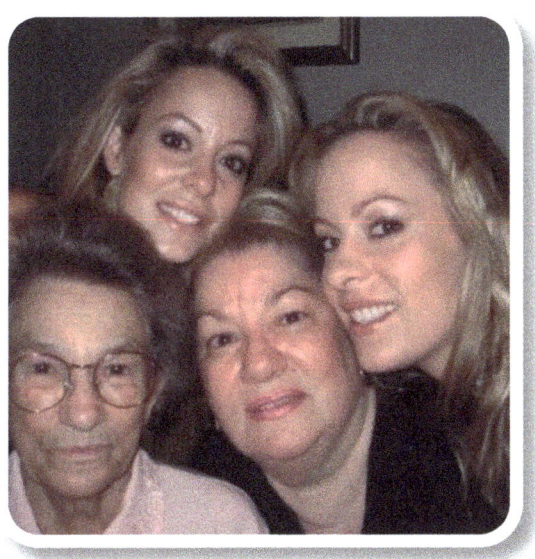

Grandma, Nicole, Mum, and Amanda

during rehabilitation and later broadened my perspective of my recovery for the long haul. It has been, and still is, an ongoing journey of maintenance.

Thank you to my friends and everyone who has been in my life since, supporting and loving me on my journey. As I finish this book, which has taken me nearly 5 years to complete, I celebrate 14 years of clear MRIs, no disease progression and a remission.

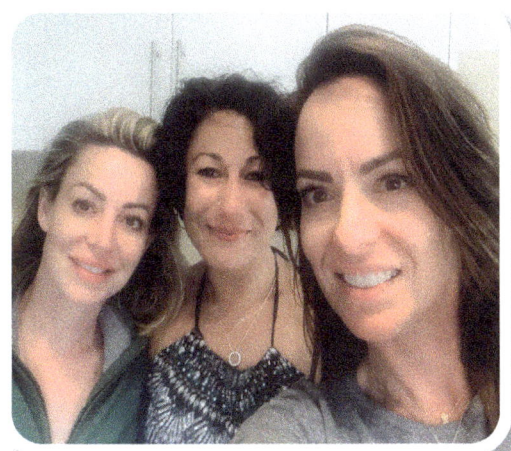

Nicole, Anthea & Amanda

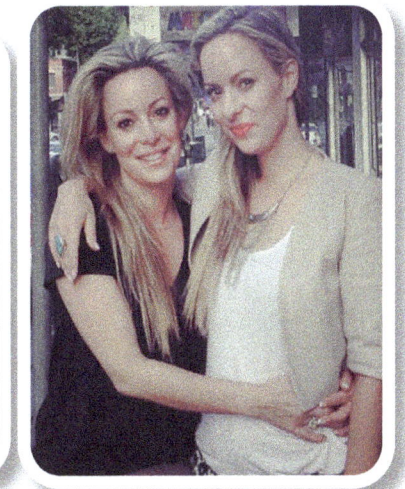

Nicole and Amanda together

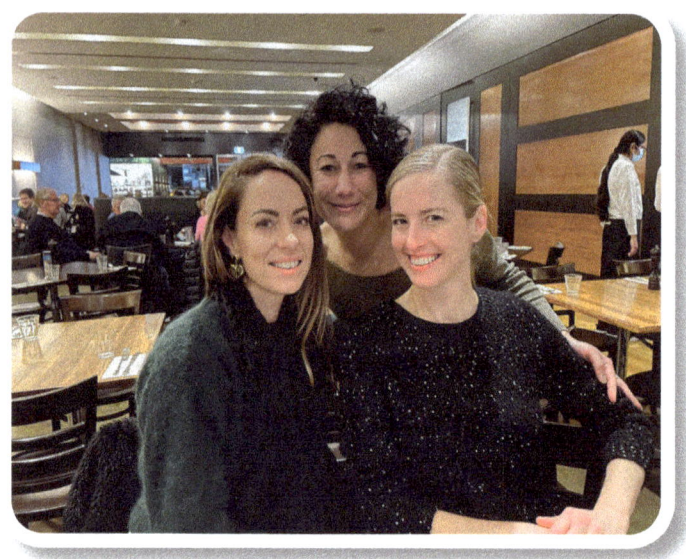

Amanda, Anthea & Bianca

The importance of seeking joy

After my toe moved for the first time, I felt hope. This created more positive thoughts – feelings of joy – rejuvenating my willpower. It renewed my mindset. As a result, I changed how I perceived my environment and how I saw my circumstances. The most fascinating part of all was witnessing how my body responded to the shifts in my mind.

It was like my body mirrored my mind. I noticed that I started to repair faster, and I began to experience how connected our minds and bodies are. Just like a tensegrity structure[47], everything works together synergistically.

I believe joy and gratitude are states that can help us to promote growth and repair pathways. I know that when I am in a joyful state of gratitude, I am so much more creative,

---

47 - Tensegrity, or tensile integrity, describes a system of isolated, compressed components within a network of chords that are under continuous tension. In a pure tensegrity structure, these components do not touch but experience compression nonetheless.

and solution-focused. Amazing things happen on the days whe I can access more joy. It feels like I'm in sync, on path, swimming downstream.

For many people, receiving and letting in joy and pleasure may have been blocked as a form of protection or punishment. There are many different reasons why we block joy; it could be self-sabotage, from fear, or because it is familiar to be in the hustle of a fight or flight state, taking life seriously and not allowing for any fun time. It can also be a mirror image of a belief that life is not working out for us. When we receive joy into our mind, body and life, it is relaxing, which is very healing. Trusting and believing that great things are possible in our lives is critical for our mental wellbeing.

When I went out for dinner with my girlfriends on the night my toe moved for the first time, I felt so happy and grateful for the experience of just being in the moment with my friends. For some reason, that night I let joy flow into my heart, and I felt it absorb into my cells. It felt like I was experiencing joy for the first time in a new way. Biochemically, emotionally and spiritually, it was an experience I will never forget.

Adversities are generally followed by joy. We live in a world of polarity, so perhaps joy is only really understood after we have known the depths of despair. Maybe that is how we should view adversity, as an event we must overcome, to stretch, learn and grow. That is why it is so important to know how to regulate our stress levels and emotions, so that we can better equipped to choose who we want to be in each moment. There is a ripple effect from each choice we make.

After my joyful experience with the girls, my toe moved for the first time and that ended up being the catalyst for me to be able to shift what I was believing about what could be possible for me. I felt guided, more held than I ever had before. Living in rehab and learning how to walk again was one of the hardest things I have ever had to do. But it was also the best time of my life, as I was forced to go within and found access to a guidance and power that remains with me today. I felt totally held, despite lying there alone surrounded by 4 white walls. In the silence, I learned how to listen to an inner knowing that everything was okay. This guidance is always there for us; but to access it, we must learn how to be idle and still. I can forget to do this if I do not consciously think about it; that is why I find a daily ritual is so important.

I now practise getting myself into an anchored and flexible state at the start and end of every day, with a journaling and meditation ritual. This is followed by my program of mind, body, food and connection rituals. Letting more joy into my life helps me to be more open to change, to be more creative and to feel more connected. This state alters the decisions I make and how I show up in the world. Mastering flexibility in my mind, I can let go of how I think things should happen; I can go with the flow in life, and it feels more like a fun adventure.

Can you choose joy, despite chaos and change? What can you do to bring you joy? What opens your heart? There is magic in feeling and receiving joy.

Henry

When I came home from hospital in 2009, a gift came to into my life exactly when I needed it. A little ray of sunshine! On Christmas Eve, nine months after I'd come home from hospital, I bought an adorable black baby pug. I named him Henry, and he kissed and cuddled me through my recovery and beyond. There were some great days when having him by my side was wonderful to share, and there were more difficult days when he would snuggle extra close because he just knew. He became another reason to get up and keep fighting on the harder days.

I had never experienced such love and connection with an animal before. Henry opened my heart to love again and helped me reconnect back to my heart in ways I never had before, the very ingredient that would lead to immense healing within me. I became a mum for the first time. Looking after a little being was the best thing for me, after being taken care of by my loving family for so long.

Henry passed away on the 10th November 2021 just after his 12th birthday, and joined my Mum on the other side only 6 months after she passed away. That was a very difficult year for me and my family.

Eva my fur daughter has since come into my life and has literally brought me back to life, hence the name Eva meaning 'life'. Her birthday is the day after Henry's x

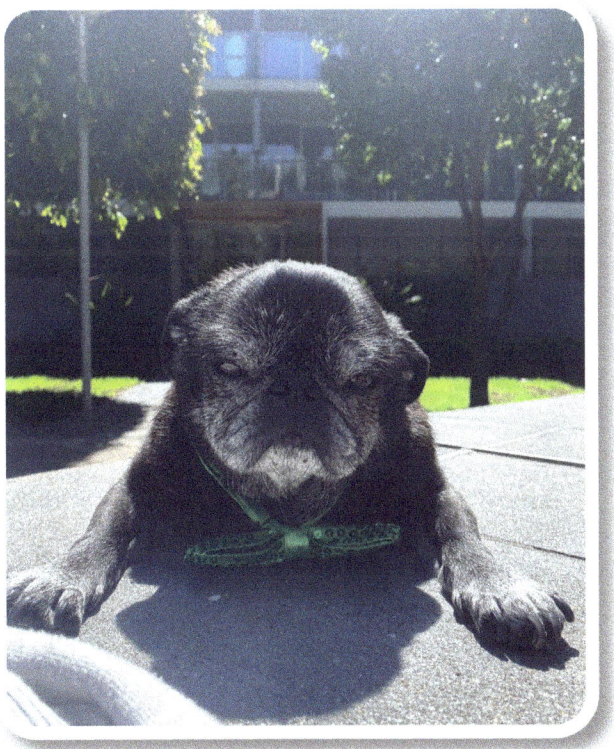

Henry

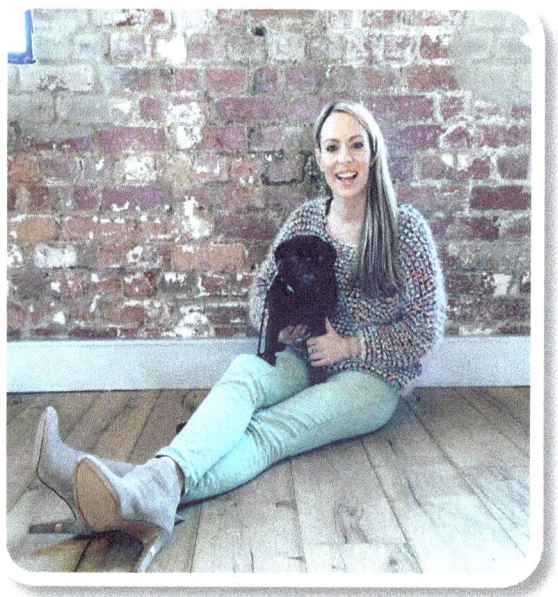

Henry with Amanda work at Nourissh

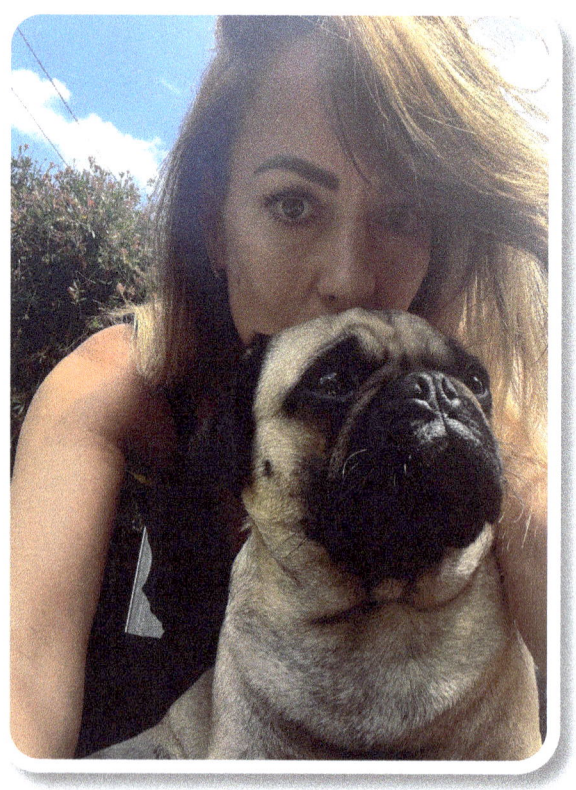

Amanda and her baby girl Eva

A new me and a new career

My recovery inspired me to go back to college to study Sports Kinesiology at the Australian College of Complementary Medicine, so I could learn Chinese medicine and the mind-body connection. It was an intense few years' study, but I persisted and met a great tribe of people who believed in me and opened my mind to the power of kinesiology.

While I was studying, it was fascinating to connect the dots in my recovery. I had an introduction into Sports Science, learning about the anatomy, physiology and motor learning of the body, entwined with the emotional and energetic philosophy of traditional Chinese medicine. It made so much sense to me. We learned that how you think and feel plays a huge role in inflammation, disease and recovery. We learned and worked on multiple cases of diseases, anxiety, depression, body pain, corrective exercise, nutrition and fertility. I learned how to apply mindset, movement and nutrition into an integrated and customised program for my clients.

One of my best mates, Bianca Millar, had given me a few flyers to study kinesiology and one stood out: Australian College of Complementary Medicine. I remember the day I rang the school and one of the owners, Carl Montgomery, answered the phone. His optimism and knowledge sparked my attention immediately. Carl developed the Diploma of Sports Kinesiology, which fuses the modality of kinesiology with sports science. Carl taught me what kinesiology can do for the body structurally. This intrigued me, as I wanted to further understand the physical mechanics of the body (fascia, tendons, ligaments, nerves, muscles, bones) and their links to our emotional wellbeing. This also helped me to dive deeper into understanding the process of how I walked again, after I recovered from my paralysis. Carl was a fantastic lecturer, he pushed me hard but lovingly. This course changed my life and set me on a new career direction.

An old friend, Nicole Papasavas, came with me to the open day, helping me to decide whether this new career approach was the right move for me. My mates, who knew me well, thankfully guided me to lean into such a dramatic career change – from fashion to wellness. The government at the time subsidised part of the cost of the course. It all made sense, so I decided to go back to school and study for a few years.

I remember when I walked up to the reception desk and told Glenda that I was quitting. I did this twice. It was so much work and, on some days, I didn't know how I was going to get all my assignments done. I'll never forget the day Carl said, with a sparkle in his eye, that he believed I was going to do something very special in my career and with kinesiology. I remember the day of my graduation, when Carl handed me my diploma, and the joy I felt after two years of hard work and dedication. I thank Carl for believing in me, even when I didn't at times.

I am so grateful to have had the opportunity to study at the college with the talented teachers I had. I made amazing friends there too, some who I still see today. Thank you to the beautiful souls who touched me in some way; I have mentioned many of you in the Acknowledgements at the end of this book.

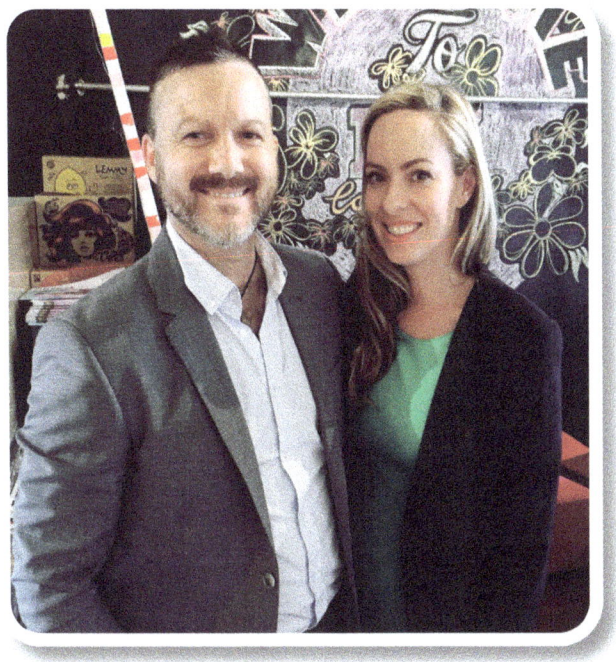

Amanda & Mike Rowan, Osteopath, Naturopath, Acupuncturist and now dear friend. Total Health Osteo in Prahran was my first location for Bend Like Bamboo in 2013.

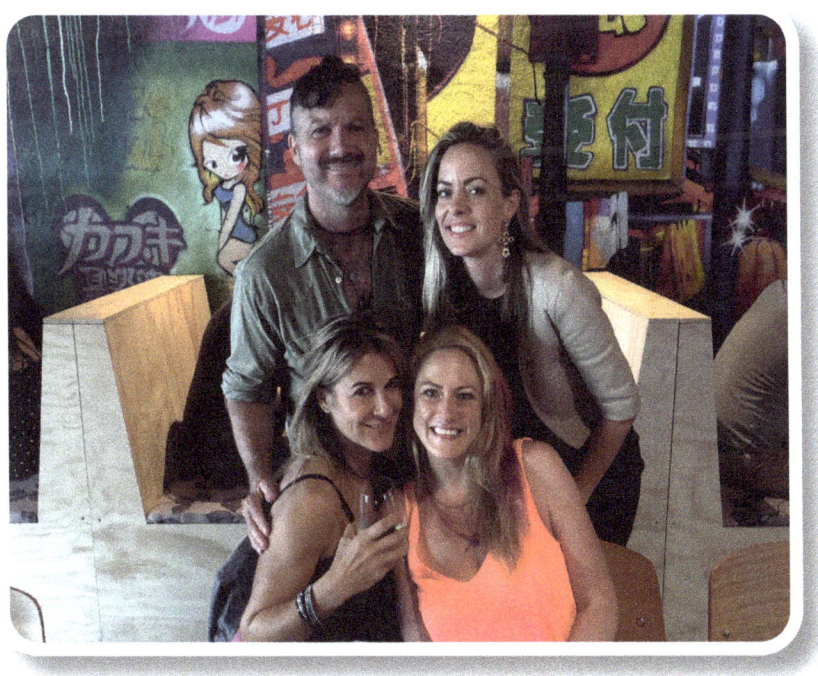

Mike, Amanda, Peggy and Nina at our work Christmas party

I graduated with my diploma at the start of 2013 and began practising in a room at my twin sister's beauty salon at the time, *Nicole's Body Boutique* in Camberwell. It was so much fun being in the same space as my twin. However, the room was very small and I wanted to expand with my own wings, so I started to look for the perfect space to call home.

That is how I met my dear friend, Mike Rowan. He is also a twin who practises as a naturopath, osteopath and acupuncturist. His business is called *Prahran Health Osteo*. I was sitting across from it having a drink at *Babble Bar & Cafe*, after a day of looking at many other spaces. I saw a for lease sign on his window and knocked on the door. In between clients, he welcomed me in for a chat and I just knew in my heart that I had found my space.

I explained that I was a new practitioner looking for a room to grow my practice; he met Henry, who ended up coming to work with me every day, and the rest is history. Mike is such a beautiful soul and a talented healer. I am so glad we met and am so grateful for his love and generosity; he gave me an opportunity to grow slowly in his space, accommodating me right from the start, supporting me all the way. I shared my room at times with an amazing soul and psychologist, Peggy Kardaras. Both Peggy and Mike have grown to become my work family and beautiful friends that I love so much.

I was able to fund the cost of opening my company, *Bend Like Bamboo*, with the help of a Go for Gold Scholarship. My thanks to MS Plus and the 24-Hour Mega Swim, founded by my MS Mentor, Carol Cooke. I have been a proud MS Ambassador for MS Plus for over a decade now, a volunteer role I have really enjoyed.

I was lucky to have a spike in PR and media, thanks to wonderful people who encouraged me to share my story with confidence. My story went viral, initially thanks to Australia's celebrity chef, Pete Evans, who shared my story with his one million followers on Facebook. Very quickly, I began to see clients from all over the world who wanted to work with me. As a result, I became very busy at my practice in a short space of time. I have been lucky to have worked with people with various physical and mental ailments or disease, and they have all helped make me the practitioner I am now. This has allowed me to identify patterns. I began to understand the mind and body from a practitioner's point of view, as well as from that of a patient.

Today at my private practice, *Bend Like Bamboo*, I specialise in the emotional links to disease, physical stress and autoimmune disease.

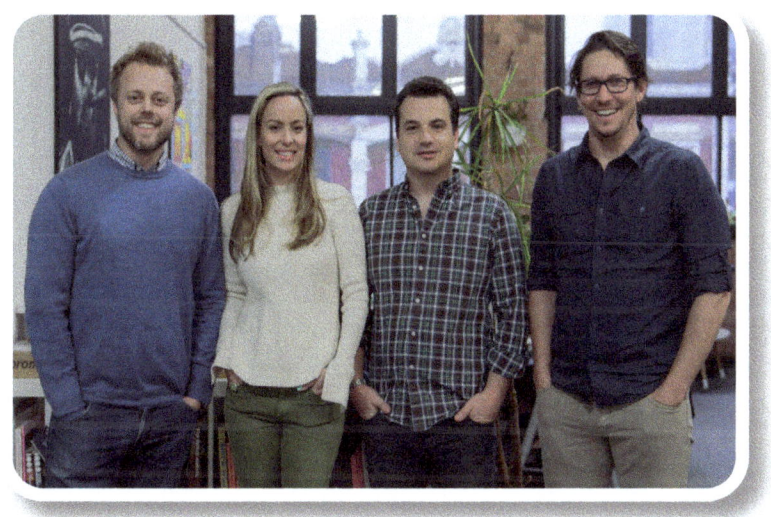

Amanda & her then partner Scott Julian, Justin Dry & Andre Eikmeier from Vinomofo who were our co-founders at Nourissh.

A year later in 2014, I co-founded *Nourissh* with investors *Vinomofo* and my partner at the time, Scott Julian. Scott and I met in 2013, just after I graduated in Sports Kinesiology. He helped me to see what could be possible for *Bend Like Bamboo*, and I will always be grateful for all the amazing adventures he brought into my life. After educating my clients about the importance of nutrition and repair at *Bend Like Bamboo*, together Scott and I saw an opportunity to go on a mission to nourish Australians on a cellular level with healthy, fresh, ready-made, wholefood meals for time poor individuals.

Nourissh became a business that focused on an innovative way of preparing and delivering healthy, sustainable, fresh, ready-made meals to individuals and businesses. On this incredible journey, I had to learn how to be on top of my game. As CEO, I had to perform in a fast-paced and innovative environment; I had to be solution-focused as my team and I were creating a re-imagined and exciting way to eat and deliver healthy and fresh meals. This is when I learned that optimising wellbeing also enhances our performance at work. Our customers were time poor from work, stress, disability and other life circumstances. I am so proud of what we achieved at *Nourissh*. We were building a new innovative food and technology business. I knew I had to see our obstacles from the 'mountain peak', where I was able to access more creative solutions with an elevated mindset through all the challenges that we faced. This was one of the best things I have done, and I am so grateful for the opportunity.

This is when I met my dear friend, Gina Lutz who applied to work in at our HQ at *Nourissh*. Navigating the highs and lows of a start-up led to a close bond and friendship. Gina is the kindest and most loyal person who is still a big part of my life.

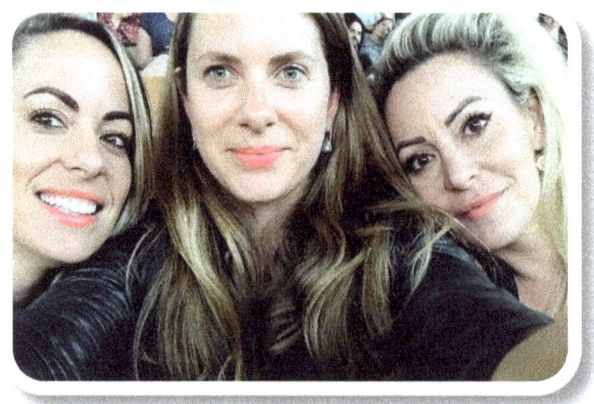

Amanda, Gina and Nicole

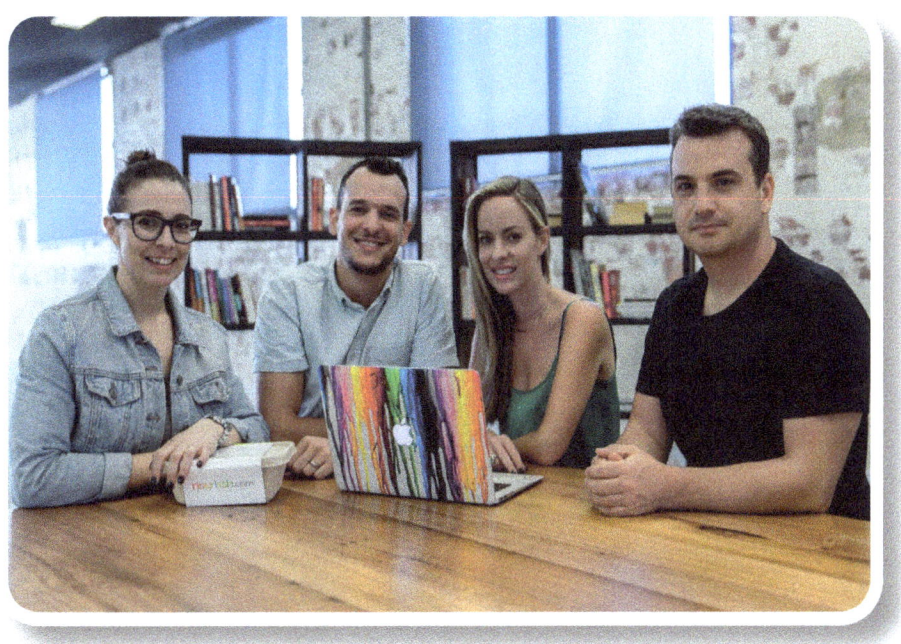

Erin, Mehdi, Amanda & Scott some of the Nourissh H/O crew

I believe that no matter what you are going through, know that life is all about cycles and phases. I have learned that there is a time when amazing opportunities come in that can open up your life in ways you never had expected. It is a wonderful time of growth and sometimes success. We cannot predict them, and we cannot force them to happen. There is also a time for stillness and reflection, a phase of preparation for what is to come next. Believe in possibility and anchor into the phase you are in on your cycle of life. My Mum would always say to me "darling, every day when you wake up, something incredible can always happen."

What if I fall?
Oh, but my darling, what if you fly?
Erin Hanson, Australian poet

Chapter 13

Reassessing Goals

In the Goal Setting exercise (Chapter 10), you wrote down a goal that you wanted to achieve. Think about that goal and ask yourself the following 3 questions:

1. What is your desire or goal?
2. What is the fear you were wanting to overcome?
3. With a flexible mindset, have you been able to change your mind about what you believe about yourself, your circumstances, and what is possible for you?

Now think about the positive beliefs you wrote about yourself, your worth, and your ability to achieve your goal. You wrote this opposite your goal on the top right side of the paper. Further down the page, you wrote down any negative or limiting beliefs you might have had about your ability to achieve your goal, or why it may not be possible for you. Have a think about that now and review what you have written.

Keep up the good work; this is a journey that will evolve day by day. If you can live your life creating, rather than reacting, you can take on anything. This is a lifestyle shift. May your new daily routines help you to heal, grow and evolve into the highest version of yourself you can possibly imagine.

Go within and ask yourself: Do I feel a shift? Perhaps bringing this information into your awareness has brewed up some stuff, and that is okay. Trust that your body knows what to do, to reorganise the chaos.

I recommend having support through this time, with a trusted practitioner who is right for you, who can help you process anything that may have come up for you. I hope that the concepts and ideas shared in my book have brought more awareness of what has been holding you back, have helped you to believe in yourself, and that an introduction to the tools is helpful for you.

Further resources on all these tools can be found in the Appendix and Reference chapters at the end of this book and on my website.

A rebuild of my mind, body and life

For every adversity, there is an equal or greater opportunity. After living in rehabilitation for two months, I was finally mobile again and able to go home. I was back in the same house, same environment, but everything looked totally different. I had grown and evolved so much from what I had gone through and was seeing my world with new eyes. It looked so beautiful; I saw evidence of beauty in the simple things. This experience brought even more joy into my heart. Different things mattered to me now. I was so grateful to be mobile again, but for a while I still had to lie down for half of every day. I suffered from new MS symptoms that were debilitating on my more difficult days, and I felt emotionally lost. So I had to rebuild myself, emotionally and physically.

My confidence took a hit for several months, while I was relying on others to help me with the most basic tasks. Being an independent person, it was difficult having to cope with needing so much help. This forced me to learn how to receive help openly and joyfully, which turned out to be exactly what I needed to heal from very old wounds. Receiving kindness and compassion from the people around me opened my heart. I had unforgettable and incredibly beautiful moments with friends and family who fed me, bathed and dressed me in my most vulnerable moments. I will never forget how deeply their love touched my heart.

But the ongoing recovery was brutal. As the weeks and months wore on, I fell into deep sadness; it felt like I had lost my old self. Rebuilding at home for the next year was sometimes harder than what I had experienced in hospital, when I couldn't walk. It was scary, lonely and confusing.

Lose what needs to be lost, to find what needs to be found.

This is a quote I love from the movie, *E-Motion*[48]. For me, it means that we need to lose sight of the shore to discover new oceans and aspects of ourselves. Old parts need to die off for us to rediscover who we are and what we are made of. The loss is what leads to our awakening.

Mum articulated the loss of confidence within me very well. She said, 'It was like I had lost the swing in my stride.' She was right.

I started on a new medication that required me to inject myself four times a week – three times more than the previous drug. This new medication led to side effects that made my body puffy, and I gained nearly 10 kilos in 3 months. I am an identical twin and have a petite frame, so this weight gain and fluid retention made me unrecognisable, at least to myself. A few years later, I saw a video of me during that time and asked my sister, 'Hey, who is that on the couch?' She kindly replied, 'That is you!' I was blown away, as I didn't recognise myself.

I was grateful to be mobile, but I knew deep within that there was still more work to be done. I went on a quest to find stories of other people who had recovered from illness or paralysis and began researching the concept of rapid recovery. This led me to discover stories of others who had recovered from MS, and I began to understand that the outcome was not the same for everyone. In fact, each case is unique in how the symptoms presented and how recovery played out. I wanted to understand why. What

---

48 - https://www.e-motionthemovie.com/

was at play here? I hit the books and researched; it became my mission to understand the mind-body connection and how to maximise repair.

When I was paralysed, I had a new lesion on the motor skill area of my brain, which was very serious. While learning more about recovery, I discovered that we have the best chance of walking again if we can have immediate, aggressive neuro-physiotherapy, as soon as possible after a stroke, brain injury or MS relapse. The first few weeks and months are critical for recovery.

I know that I was very lucky with my recovery. Perhaps I was in the right place at the right time, surrounded by the right people, in the right environment, with the right amount of determination and the right mindset for the magic to happen. Maybe there was also a higher force at play? Sometimes these things are not able to be explained and we don't fully know why. I am just so grateful, and I see my recovery as a second chance at my life.

Going through my illness taught me valuable lessons. Understanding MS from a practitioner's perspective, as well as a patient's, helps me to have more compassion for my clients, and this is why people living with autoimmune disease come and see me.

Rebuilding from loss and grief

I have learned that, in life, there are going to be a number of times when we will have to rebuild ourselves. In 2021, Mum died on Mother's Day, very suddenly in my arms. My heart was completely broken. Only six months later, my fur baby Henry died in my arms from a stroke, totally unexpectedly. My heart was now shattered and in pieces; it unravelled me. All the walls that I had spent much of my life building around my heart to protect me, now had no choice but to fall down. This experience was excruciating and so difficult to go through.

At that time, I was also rebuilding my life after a separation. I had to learn how to be there for myself, when I didn't have my family at home to support me in moments of complete despair. I understand now why this process had to happen, the grief was so intense for me. I had to let go of the old me who learned how to be tough and strong; the grief forced me to access vulnerability, a feeling that was very triggering for me. I had to rebirth a totally new version of myself that could let go, rebuild and heal with a quieter mind, an open heart, patience and more discipline. A whole new dimension of having to bend like bamboo is before me and I am learning more and more every day as I heal on this journey.

Where I am now

2023 marked my fourteenth year of clear MRIs, and every year keeps getting better and better. I continue to work with a great team; their approach is to reverse engineer my disease. I have found it be effective to connect the degeneration to the systems of my body and its pathways. Our goal is to get to the cause of inflammation and stress and, in my case, the end result that we call MS. I have loved specialists such as kinesiologists, naturopaths, nutritionists, acupuncturists, functional trainers and functional medical practitioners, neuro-physiotherapists and neurologists. In my experience, I found it really helpful to have a great GP who supports my balanced approach.

What maximised my recovery was not just one thing. It has been a personal journey with a lot of help from various people who I have had the privilege to work with along the way. This continues in my current maintenance program.

Taking a balanced approach has helped me to cover the broad range of moving parts that I believe contribute to optimising wellness. I have an incredible neurologist, who takes the time to listen to my questions; she supports my initiative to be proactive and my balanced approach. I utilise Western medicine and medications that have been right for me, particularly in times of acute and immediate intervention. I also combine the Western approach with an Eastern one, and that has helped me to evaluate my thinking, nutrition and movement habits.

I believe that conventional medicine works well in conjunction with natural medicine. I've found that educating myself about the various fields of repair and recovery has empowered me and made me become an active and informed patient, reaping benefits from all approaches available in the field of medicine. Knowledge is power and only improves patient care. I do hope we can soon live in a world where doctors teach and educate their clients about wellness prevention and dealing with the cause of their disease, as well as treating their symptoms with conventional drugs.

Because I have created the momentum in optimising my wellbeing, I now enjoy a maintenance health program that aids prevention and keeps me accountable. The tools and strategies I have learned helps me to process life every day. I live life more aware and awake; I can manage stress better, I attract more amazing opportunities and, most importantly, I feel happy and well.

Life guided me to move to the Mornington Peninsula in 2022 and I have loved living by the sea. It has been very healing to be emersed in nature, deepening my inner anchor as I explore this next chapter in my 40's. Eva my furbaby and I are on a new adventure, and I am enjoying becoming a new version of myself that enjoys striving less and the simplicity in life.

I hope my book inspires you to believe in yourself. With the power of flexibility, we can heal, we can grow and overcome with more ease. Loving ourselves a little bit more can enable us to promote self-care and prevention.

I believe that illness, setbacks and changes in life are there to help us grow; as we push ourselves out of our comfort zone more and more, we realise how resilient we are and what we are truly made of. This realisation brings joy and an inner anchor within us. I believe this is the best environment we can give ourselves to rise above our setbacks, to transform our obstacles into opportunities, and to believe in ourselves. All the lessons we learn along the way build resilience and confidence within us, so that we can realise our fullest potential in this life. Obstacles are opportunities and detours towards the next best path for you. You are supposed to feel uncomfortable, otherwise you'd just stay the same. If we are not open to change and are feeling rigid from stress, we cannot see these moments that I believe are miracles that can change our lives for the better.

There is no quick fix, this is a journey. If you are ready for change, start with your mind, with what you are thinking, saying and believing. Once you can become more flexible you may notice a shift, and this transformation will translate into your body, your love life, your work life and within all your relationships.

When you really believe in yourself, others will believe in you too. It all starts with you and building your inner anchor. We all have the tools and resources we need inside of us to repair and transform our lives.

When life throws the bigger curve balls and change, remember that you are on an exceptional journey. Don't compare it to anyone else's, we are all on our own timeline. There is a time for loss and a time for a comeback too! Never give up, Mr Edison tried 10,000 combinations before he learned to 'tune in' to his inner anchor and intuition that led him to get the answer that perfected the incandescent light.

I hope you feel inspired to change your mind about what can be possible in your mind, body and life. Thank you for your valuable time and for listening to my story and the lessons I've learned along the way. I am honoured to share them with you. And welcome to the Bend Like Bamboo family. You are loved and supported, your journey is special.

No matter what you are going through, I believe that you can overcome it and discover just how powerful you really are. This is the art of Bending Like Bamboo: reimagining what can be possible, rising to our challenges with courage and resilience. It is our ability to return to our inner anchor, where we can choose to reconnect and relax through life's experiences. This is the space where miracles happen, where our superpower is revealed, where we can let go of the world as we knew it, and step into a new realm of possibility.

May the force be with you x

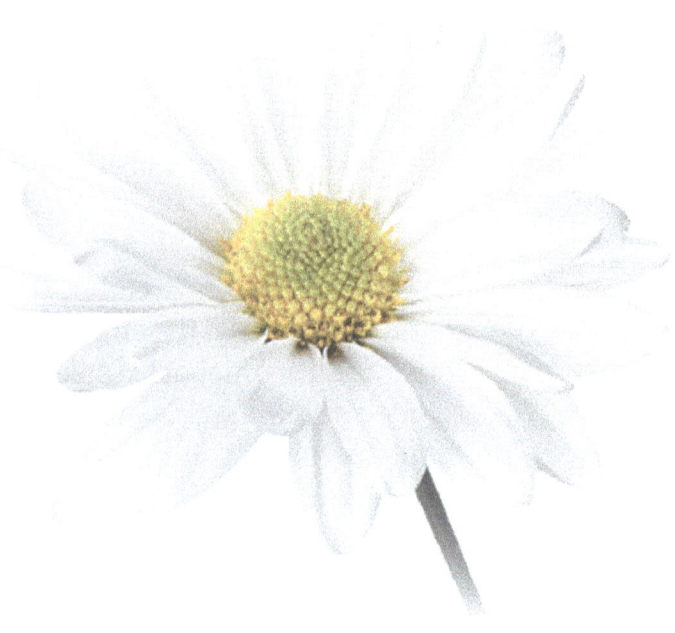

About the Author

In 2013, Amanda founded *Bend Like Bamboo* her private practice. As a trained Sports Kinesiologist Amanda specialises in Multiple Sclerosis & Autoimmune Disease, helping individuals to destress to heal their minds, bodies, and lives. *Bend Like Bamboo* has since evolved to become a wellness program. As a resilience trainer, and keynote speaker, she works with leaders, athletes, and kids, helping them to master resilience, and uncover blind spots to achieve their personal and professional goals. How does she do this? Amanda teaches people how to Bend Like Bamboo.

After her own diagnosis of Multiple Sclerosis at age 24 and overcoming a left-hand side body paralysis at age 29, her journey led to discovering an inner anchor within that allowed her to adapt. Helping others she has discovered that a flexible mindset impacts everything that matters: our body's ability to repair, how happy and resilient we can be and our ability to reach our fullest potential. Amanda is not only the practitioner, but also the patient which allows her to have a deeper understanding of the challenges her clients face, living with an autoimmune disease.

Amanda believes that with a flexible mindset we can build resilience, and building resilience improves our well-being. Available in-person and online, The Bend Like Bamboo program is customisable for individuals, schools, and workplaces around Australia & globally.

In 2014, Amanda co-found *Nourissh* with Scott Julian and *Vinomofo*, a business that focused on an innovative way of preparing and delivering healthy, sustainable, fresh, ready-made meals to individuals and businesses.

Amanda is also an MS Ambassador, a volunteer role she has enjoyed as a speaker since 2009, when she first learned how to share her story to spread awareness and to help others.

Appendix

Contact info

Bend Like Bamboo resilience blog and podcast
    Blog: https://www.amandacampbell.com.au/blog
    Podcast: https://www.amandacampbell.com.au/podcasts
    YouTube: https://www.youtube.com/user/BendLikeBamboo

www.amandacampbell.com.au
    Workplace Resilience Program
    School Resilience Program
    Keynote Speaking & Workshops
    Online Courses
    Corporate Retreats

www.bendlikebamboo.com
    Sports Kinesiology
    Online Courses
    Retreats

Socials

Amanda Campbell

FB: www.facebook.com/amandacampbellspeaker

IG: www.instagram.com/amandacampbell_speaker/

Twitter: twitter.com/AmandaC_health

LinkedIn: www.linkedin.com/in/amandacampbellau

Bend Like Bamboo

FB: www.facebook.com/BendLikeBamboo

IG: www.instagram.com/bendlikebamboo/

Bend Like Bamboo and the Anatomy of Resilience

B — Being with ourselves, creating space in our daily lives for quiet time, personal space to reflect, regularly checking in with our higher self and guidance. Quietening the mind allows a deeper connection within ourselves, filling our cup, so we can connect more with our tribe. Schedule this time in your diary, as you would a meeting.

E — Exercise your body with stretches and exercise. Movement is a great way to build strength and endurance, promoting fitness and gut health. Movement is another way to elevate our mindset, boosting emotional resilience.

N — Nourish yourself on a cellular level. Every meal is an opportunity to nourish ourselves, promoting repair. Food is fuel and information for our cells, which require nutrients to perform and heal. When we eat better, we feel better, allowing us to be more adaptable and resilient.

D — Do something that scares you every day! This is a great way to get out of your comfort zone, stretching your limits, proving to yourself what you are capable of. When the bigger challenges come, you will be ready.

L   **L**ove yourself, be your own best friend. How can you give what you have not learned to create and be for yourself? Loving yourself is reflected in the choices we make, our inner dialogue and, inevitably, how happy and healthy we are.

I   **I**ndividualise your own path forward, be brave enough to pave your own way, walking a road that creates the life you desire and aligns with what brings you joy.

K   **K**ill off negativity and the monkey mind, old beliefs, narratives, judgements and negative emotions that hold you back. Create space for the new to come into your life.

E   **E**levate your mindset to access more elevated emotions: kindness, courage, love, forgiveness. What we think, feel and believe all use energy. Battling with our inner conflicts and feeling the inner resistance within that holds us back, all consume energy. When we can begin to believe in ourselves and what can be possible for us, a shift and alignment occurs; we begin to focus on what we want, on the positive, and we feel hope. Receiving more joy and hope in our lives re-energises our mind, body and soul.

B	**B**ecoming a new version of ourselves is a transformation that requires …
A	**A**mbition. Want your goal more than whatever anchors you into your suffering and keeps you stuck.
M	**M**imic people who inspire you. There's no need to reinvent the wheel, it can be valuable to research and explore proven models that already work and take inspiration from them.
B	**B**uild a new mindset, thoughts, habits and story. Putting one foot in front of the other may seem incremental and slow, but having the intention to do something every single day towards your goal leads you to your destination faster than you think.
O	**O**pen your heart and choose joy despite adversity. It is the best environment you can give yourself to optimise repair and performance.
O	**O**bstacles are your opportunity to grow and heal. The lessons you are learning as you go through setbacks, change and adversity are helping you to grow and become a new version of yourself. The more flexible and adaptable you can be in the process, the more enjoyable the ride will be.

References

A full resource library of references and free resources can also be found on my website: www.bendlikebamboo.com

Research articles and references

Neuroanatomy reticular activating system – www.ncbi.nlm.nih.gov, 2023

Study Guide to the Systems of the Body – Amanda Menard, LPN, 2017

Brain Cells that Suppress Fear Memories Hide in the Hippocampus, Neuroscience Research, University of Texas at Austin, 2019

Women Have More Active Brains Than Men—MedicalXpress.com, 2017

Cerebral cavernous malformations: from CCM genes to endothelial cell homeostasis—PubMed, 2013

The role of the hypothalamic-pituitary-adrenal axis in neuroendocrine responses to stress—ncbi.nlm.nih.gov, 2006

Applying a system approach to thyroid physiology: Looking at the whole with a mitochondrial perspective instead of judging single TSH values or why we should know more about mitochondria to understand metabolism—www.ncbi.nlm.nih.gov, 2017

Human Microbiome Project—National Institutes of Health, 2017

Amygdala activity predicts post-traumatic stress disorder—AlphaGalileo, 2017

Connections found between each meridian & organ representation area of corresponding internal organs in each side of the cerebral cortex—PubMed, 1989

References

Science finally proves meridians exist—Uplift, 2016

Estimating the accuracy of muscle response testing—BMC, 2016

Your Unconscious Mind Is Running Your Life

Effect of negative emotions on frequency of coronary heart disease—The Normative Ageing Study, The American journal of cardiology, 2003

Emotional intelligence, life satisfaction and subjective happiness in female student health professionals: the mediating effect of perceived stress, https://pubmed.ncbi.nlm.nih.gov/23578272/ Pub Med, John Wiley & Sons Ltd, 2013

https://newsroom.uhc.com/health/writing-wellness.html#:~:text=Research%2C%20while%20still%20ongoing%2C%20has,adapt%20and%20feel%20less%20overwhelmed, United Healthcare, 2020

National Centre for Integrative and Integrative Health, https://www.nccih.nih.gov/health/meditation-in-, depth#:~:text=Many%20studies%20have%20investigated%20meditation,may%20help%20people%20with%20insomnia, 2022

https://www.msaustralia.org.au/news/exercise-and-ms/

Mindset specialists

The following are referenced throughout the book:

Bruce Lipton, American developmental biologist

Dr. Joe Dispenza, researcher on neuroscience, epigenetics and mindset

Wayne Dwyer, motivational speaker and author

Anita Moorjani, author and speaker

Caroline Myss – Myss.com

Marissa Peer.com

John E. Sarno

Dr Libby Weaver – https://www.drlibby.com/

More free resources, articles and studies can be found at www.bendlikebamboo.com

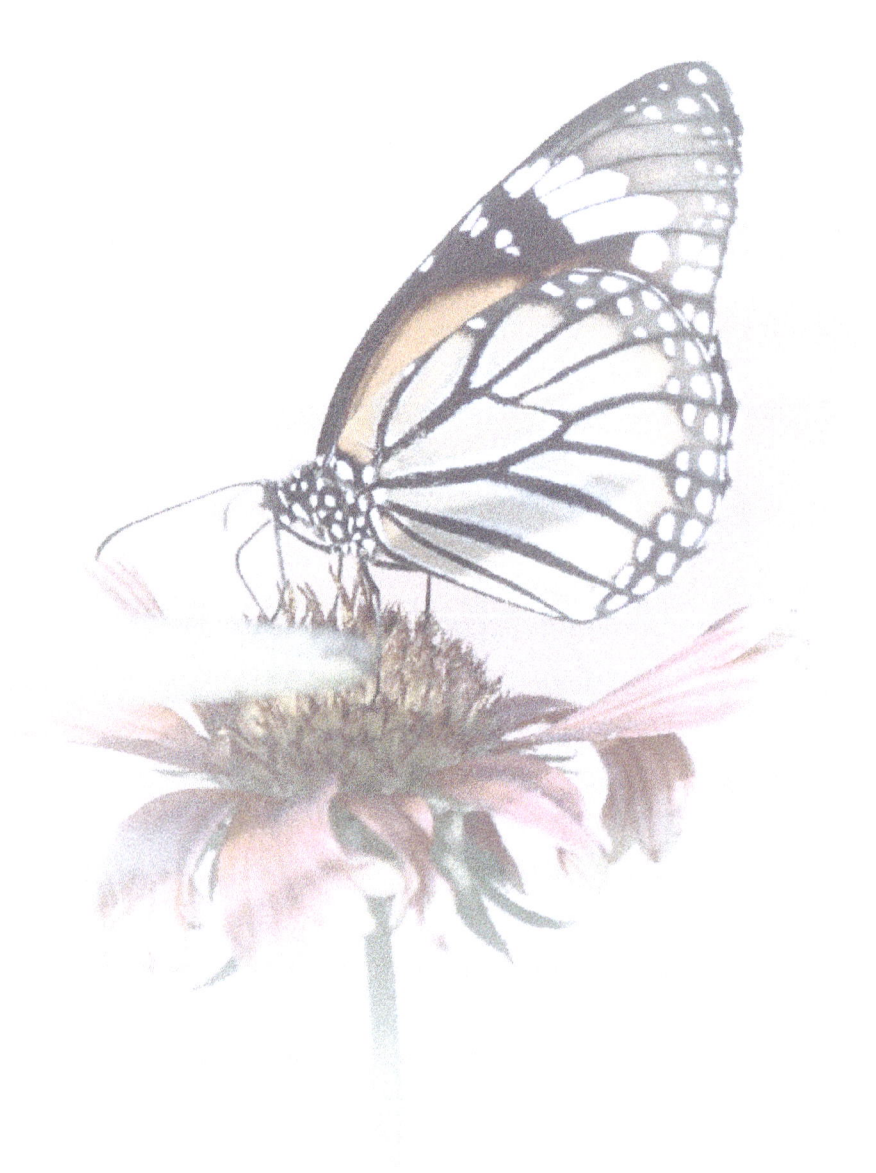

Acknowledgements

My recovery wasn't just about me, far from it. I had an amazing team of people who helped me, and who helped me believe that I could do it. They stood with me when I couldn't stand and helped me along the journey. I'd like to take the time to acknowledge the Eastern and Western doctors, family, friends and colleagues that have been an integral part of my recovery and *Bend Like Bamboo*.

Family

I could not have come through this ordeal with courage and determination, if it had not been for my loving supportive family and friends – in particular, my twin sister, Nicole. She was there for me day and night when I was paralysed; I count my lucky stars for her love and compassion through the hardest time of my life.

Thank you to my Mum, Muma and Dad, for loving me and educating us, and for doing your best. Families aren't perfect, but I know we all love each other very deeply and I thank my parents for all the wonderful opportunities they provided for Nicole and me.

My Mum has since left this planet on Mother's Day, 9 May 2021, and I dedicate this book to her. My Mum always loved me and never judged me. No matter what, I always felt so loved by you Ma, and you inspire me to push myself to keep going, to become my fullest potential and to make you proud of who I am and what I am yet to become.

Because you loved me, I know real unconditional love. I still feel your love, even though you are not physically here.

Thank you to Claire, my half-sister, for assisting Mum in hospital in her final weeks. Thank you Louise Bath and Chester Bear for flying down.

Thanks to Aunty Nada, Uncle Panda & Carol Burns for looking after me at the beach, and love to my family in Croatia Marko and Zdenka Blazevic, *volim te*.

Friends

While I was living in hospital, all the love and support really accelerated my healing. A massive thank you to all my friends for being there with me through one of the most difficult times I have ever navigated. It touched my heart and gave me the hope to keep going.

Thank you to Bianca Millar – BB – for editing my scrips, and for helping me find my kinesiology course; thank you to Matt Gdanitz for shooting my online program, your professionalism, and for making the big day so much fun. To Mimi for being like a second Mum to me, thank you for your love and guidance. Thanks to Nicole Papasavas for coming to the open day with me and encouraging me to study again.

To a very special group of mates: Vicky Marcoulis, Penny Scott, Sarah Welk, Caz Skudar, Jane Carrodus, Teisha Lowry, Daz Cox, Christine Ward, Allan and Loz Bennetto. I will always hold you in my heart; thank you for making me laugh so much and for all the visits in hospital. It meant a lot and helped me more than you know.

Nicole my sister, Nina Rossi, Anthea Michaels and Caz took turns looking after me to wash, dress and feed me. Thank you. Christine and Nick Zotos, Tina, Christopher and Tanelle Gillette, Kathy Agoos, Michelle and Valerie for your love and support – you are like family to me.

Acknowledgements

Thank you, Nicole Zurlolo, for massaging me when I was in so much pain; Bec who came into hospital to do my nails, helping me to feel better; and Annie Forrest for your love and understanding through life.

Thank you to all my friends who visited me during my 2-month stay in rehabilitation. It touched my heart and gave me hope to keep going. All your love and support really accelerated my healing, and I am so grateful to everyone who came and supported me.

Thank you to Scott Julian for helping me to see what could be possible for *Bend Like Bamboo*; I will always be grateful for the amazing adventures you brought into my life.

Mike Varigos, Olivia Villani, Michelle Rowland, Tiplet, David Foote, Mike Rowan and Peggy Kardaras, Anna Hjelmstrom, Nick Roper, Courtney Cousins, Charisse Beddome, Dara Shashoua, Polly and Shaf Kahn, Gina Lutz, Neda Rahmani, Marrs Coiro, Shane Young, Dan Robertson, Jason Lawrence, the SY21 crew ... you have all made a big impact on me and I am so grateful to have you in my life.

Doctors

Thank you Ronit Bichler, Dr Lawrence Cher, Dr. Olga Skibina, and Louise Rath – your compassion and support has made such an impact on me. Thank you for taking the time to listen to my questions, and for supporting my initiative to be proactive and have a balanced approach.

Dr. Anne Money and Dr. Meg Goswami, GPs who have been part of my journey, thank you for your guidance and believing in me. I will forever be indebted to the exceptional neuro-physiotherapists at Epworth Richmond, Gavin Williams and Shaun. Thank you for helping me to walk and run again.

To Dr. Terry Wahls, the Wahls protocol was a huge part of my recovery; thank you for seeing me in Iowa USA. And thanks to the wonderful doctors all over the world who have had the courage to educate the world about the power of food as medicine.

Kinesiology family

Thank you to Carl Montgomery for your optimism and knowledge, and my Diploma of Sports Kinesiology. Thank you to Glenda, all my teachers and fellow students at the Australian College of Complementary Medicine. Thank you to kinesiologists Dr. Michael Bay, May Clarke, Damian Brown, Jacque Mooney and Charles Krebs. To my fellow kinesiologists, the Australian Institute of Kinesiology, to the amazing volunteers that run the board, thank you for dedicating your lives to a modality that is so life-changing.

Bend like Bamboo family

Thank you, Mike Rowan and Peggy Kadaris, for being my work family and for the tribe we created in Prahran Melbourne, my soul home. Mike, thanks for giving me my first room to rent at your clinic, and for all your love and support at the very start. Thank you to Jo Harrison, Olivia Villani and Michelle Rowland for nourishing *Bend Like Bamboo* when I was working at *Nourissh*.

Thank you to Sarah Lowes, Nicola Zarb, Daria Sergienko, Brian Hines, Toni Levin, Amelia Pinkard, Michelle Kennedy, Janice Kirstin, Elvie Tagum and Melissa Corazon, Apertif Agency and Positive HR for being part of my team. Thank you to Kat Barker-Smith for your kindness when I was rebuilding, thank you to Ed Chiu, FutureStudio and team for helping me to rebrand and digitalise after the pandemic.

Thank you, Deniese Cox, not only for teaching me how to make my virtual programs engaging, but for being a very special human with healing superpowers that impact me greatly.

Thank you to MS Plus and Trish Mifsud, for supporting me as an MS Ambassador where my public speaking started; to Pete Evans for sharing my story and helping people globally to find my work.

And to all my clients, it is such an honour working with you, learning about you and assisting you on your journey. Thank you for trusting and sharing your journey with me.

Nourissh family

Thank you to Scott Julian, for the journey we had and what we built together.

Gina Lutz, you are my soul sister now; thank you for your diligence and loyalty at *Nourissh*.

A huge thank you to our investors and the team at *Vinomofo*, for believing in us and our vision. Thank you to Andre Eikmeier, Justin and Rod Dry. Together we went on a mission to nourish Australians on a cellular level with healthy, fresh, ready-made, wholefood meals. I am so grateful for the opportunity I had to build this business, one of my best achievements.

To Emma and Frankie from Paleo Pure for sharing your space with us, to chefs Matt Kennedy and David Selex for all your hard work and dedication right from the start; to all the team in the office, kitchen and out on the road driving for us, you helped us to build a brand-new concept, making a big dream that had a lot of purpose and meaning into a reality, it was one of the most difficult but amazing things I have done.

Speaking

Thank you to my mentors, Mark Truelson and Laura Huxley, for your expertise and guidance as you helped me be brave and share my story; thank you to Steve Carey, Colleen Callander, and Carol Cooke for your friendship and guidance. To Barry Gallagher who helped me to come out of my shell right at the very start.

Thank you to Lisa Sweeney, CEO of Business in Heels, to Eyob Yesus from Growth Generation for supporting and collaborating with me in your wonderful communities and businesses.

Other contributors to my book

Thank you to Millie Lester and Catherine Moolenschot for helping me piece the book together at the very start; and to Margie Tubbs for editing it, not just once, but twice. Thank you to Susan Pierce for workshopping the final structure with me and making it more digestible and actionable; and to Leon at Hay House, for your kindness and support on my writing journey.

www.ingramcontent.com/pod-product-compliance
Lightning Source LLC
Chambersburg PA
CBHW041316110526
44591CB00021B/2799